Praise for *Quantum Supplements*

"Not only am I recommending *Quantum Supplements* for my clients, but I'm excited to apply the information in my own life. I've searched near and far for a chakra-based approach to nutrition, and Deanna's book is the richest and most effective tool-set I've ever seen. This is a critical handbook for anyone who wants to blend a practical approach with chakras to equal 'real energy' for life." —Cyndi Dale, author of *The Subtle Body: An Encyclopedia of Your Energetic Anatomy*

"A detailed, informative, and comprehensive reference, *Quantum Supplements* is a fascinating guide that elevates supplementation to new a level. Deanna Minich insightfully explains how the biological and physiological affects of vitamins, minerals, herbs, and other supplements influence our emotions, behavior, and subtle energy body. This enlightening and groundbreaking book is a must read for anyone interested in holistic health, supplements, and healing. Another fascinating work by Deanna Minich!" —Elise Marie Collins, author of *Chakra Tonics* and *An A–Z Guide to Healing Foods*

"*Quantum Supplements* is an absolute gem! In a time when the majority of nutrition books simply repeat the same old tired information, Deanna Minich has created a highly innovative, practical, and compelling work. Simply put, her unique blending of energy medicine, the chakra system, and clinical nutrition is found absolutely nowhere else, and significantly pushes the envelope when it comes to supplements and health. Dr. Minich seamlessly weaves together scientific fact and ancient/intuitive wisdom in a highly readable fashion. Your understanding of vitamins, minerals, and herbs will be forever changed. I consider this book a must have reference work that takes us into the future of nutrition." —Marc David, founder and director of The Institute for the Psychology of Eating, author of *Nourishing Wisdom* and *The Slow Down Diet*

D1248357

Praise for *Chakra Foods for Optimum Health*

"*Chakra Foods* is loaded with wisdom, joy, and practicality. Reading through this book provided me with many 'ah ha!' experiences. *Chakra Foods* is full of unusual and uplifting insights that one can apply to their life instantly."
—Christiane Northrup, M.D., author of *The Secret Pleasures of Menopause* and *Women's Bodies, Women's Wisdom*

"An original and outstanding work of art and science." —Kenneth Fine, M.D., founder and director of The Intestinal Health Institute

"'The missing piece,' I whispered as I read this wonderful book. How could food be confined to such mundane terms as calories, carbs, and proteins, when the mere thought of it brings forth such great emotion and spirit? A must read!"
—Adam Banning, lecturer, radio personality, functional medicine consultant, and author of *Seeing the Angel in the Mirror*

"Successfully weaving together hard science, ancient spirituality, real-life case studies, and mouth-watering recipes, *Chakra Foods* couldn't be more innovative or down to earth. Definitely destined to become a classic." —Elise Marie Collins, author of *Chakra Tonics*

Praise for *An A–Z Guide to Food Additives*

"More than a quick reference, this is the definitive guide for the health-conscious shopper." —Robert H. Lerman, M.D., Ph.D.

"Deanna Minich is the genius of nutrition, a perfect blend of spirit and science."
—Nicole Zivalich, N.D.

"I now have a trusted resource regarding the 'loaded' issue of food additives and the conflicting information about these additives in our food supply. A must for your reference library." —Barb Schiltz, M.S., R.N., C.N.

QUANTUM
Supplements

A TOTAL HEALTH *and*
WELLNESS MAKEOVER
with VITAMINS
MINERALS, *and* HERBS

Deanna M. Minich, Ph.D., C.N.

Conari Press

First published in 2010 by Conari Press,
an imprint of Red Wheel / Weiser, LLC
With offices at:
500 Third Street, Suite 230
San Francisco, CA 94107
www.redwheelweiser.com

ISBN: 978-1-57324-420-6
Library of Congress Cataloging-in-Publication Data available upon request.

Cover design by Maxine Ressler
Text design by Donna Linden
Typeset in Perpetua, Priori Sans, and RuseX0000HG
Cover photographs: lavender flowers © felinda/iStockphoto.com, blue teapot © Charles Noble/
iStockphoto.com, assorted pills and vitamins © Matej Pribelsky, pile of rubbed sage © ilmwa555/
iStockphoto.com, bowl of turmeric root © ajaykampani/iStockphoto.com, red elderberrries © catay/
iStockphoto.com

Printed in the United States of America
TS
10 9 8 7 6 5 4 3 2 1

The paper used in this publication meets the minimum requirements of the American National Stan-
dard for Information Sciences-Permanence of Paper for Printed Library Materials Z39.48-1992
(R1997).

Dedicated to the healing of the planet:
its people, animals, plants, and water

May all beings everywhere with whom we are inseparably connected, be fulfilled, awakened, liberated, and free. May there be peace in this world and throughout the entire universe, and may we all together complete the spiritual journey.

MAHAYANA PRAYER

ACKNOWLEDGMENTS

Even though I've never given birth to a child, I believe that writing a book comes pretty close. I am incredibly grateful to all involved for the opportunity to share this creation, which is really the culmination of learning, insight, and information from numerous teachers, mentors, and friends throughout my life who have formed ripples in my internal waters.

My path to chakras, health, and nutrition has been led by several incredible individuals. The teachings of Caroline Myss have served as a wellspring of inspiration for me in the past decade. I admire her courage, strength, and direct approach that enables profound spiritual concepts to take on a practical, everyday twist. Her writings on chakras and health were essential teachings for me early in my career. Patrice Connelly trained me to see and work with my own chakras and those of others. The spiritual lessons she unraveled to me became a foundation from which to continue this healing art. Cyndi Dale has been a remarkably instrumental teacher and guide, and she has helped me to unfold the future that lie awaiting for me. Char Sundust, one of the most amazing, beautiful beings I have ever met, has helped me to grow and become teacher, writer, and artist. Her hope and faith in me gave me the spark to create. I thank her for the training in the Shamanic tradition that she provided me. It has become a thread through everything I do.

In addition to the energy healers who have influenced my path, I have had the pleasure of working with mentors in nutrition, including Jeffrey Bland, Phyllis Bowen, Maria Sapuntzakis, Clare Hasler, Henkjan Verkade, Roel Vonk, Jack Kornberg, Robert Lerman, Barb Schiltz, Donna Landry, and Lyra Heller. All of you have been beyond inspirational, encouraging me to explore health and nutrition in innovative, exciting ways. Special thanks to Barb Schiltz for taking time to edit this manuscript and provide valuable feedback and to Georgia Clark for her artistic talent and creation of the illustrations in this text.

I give gratitude to the yogic tradition that I have been a part of for twenty years and to all the many teachers I have had through this time who live and teach this ancient spiritual practice. I thank Joanna Cashman for her grace and teaching gifts that have allowed me to help others with yoga.

Heartfelt thanks to my family for their bountiful gifts: my mother for her strength, faith, and dedication to healthy living; my father for his ability to love unconditionally and be engaged with the dance of life; my sister for her keen wit, empathy, and creativity; and my brother for his humility, depth, and authenticity. My partner, Mark, has been supportive of the time and space I have needed to write. He continues to teach me the power of the middle path. I love and acknowledge the three orange furry friends (Simon, Sasha, and Charlie Brown) who surrounded me with gentle purring while I was writing this book.

My agent, Krista Goering, is a bright, brilliant soul who understands this life work and does an excellent job finding the best conduit for its appearance into the world. I appreciate her diligence and passion for the work she does. Not everyone is as fortunate to have an editor like Caroline Pincus, an angel of the publishing world. Her compassionate comments and balanced approach to writing are greatly admired.

Truly, I am in awe of all the people I have met on my life path, seeking wisdom and healing within classes I've offered or within the setting of a clinic visit. Thank you for allowing me into your lives to give and receive what I could. I remain in service to you.

CONTENTS

NOTE TO READERS

This book is intended to be an introductory, informational guide and is not meant to treat, diagnose, or prescribe. This text provides information available at the time of writing. Since the research on dietary supplements is always changing, new developments will undoubtedly be revealed over time. It is the responsibility of the individual to consult with experts and current literature for future updates on vitamin, mineral, and botanical supplements that may be relevant for physical conditions, including changes in dose, duration of use, side effects, or in treating or preventing conditions, to name a few.

Additionally, please note that this book is not a comprehensive guide to all supplements that exist for all conditions. Only a select group of supplements were included. For any medical condition or symptom, always consult with a qualified physician or appropriate healthcare professional. Neither the author nor the publisher accepts any responsibility for your health or how you choose to use the information contained in this book.

Names and identifying details have also been changed to honor people's desire for confidentiality.

INTRODUCTION

I was introduced to chakras about twenty years ago when I started taking yoga classes. Their connection to the concepts of energy and vibration was particularly intriguing to me. Being an artist drawn to the intensity of colors and the healing arts, I soon realized that the chakras were a perfect marriage of the two. Since that time, I've read countless books on chakras, attended classes on chakras, painted chakras, created chakra greeting cards, and finally learned to read and interpret the chakras. Now I work with the chakras in my own daily practice and use them as a tool in working with others. Sometimes I choose not to say that I am utilizing the chakra system as a framework to helping others, simply because it's not always necessary to get trapped in the net of an unfamiliar verbiage that may require undue explanation. To make the chakra concept more accessible and modern, I have attempted to describe the chakras differently, capturing their essence for the nonsubscribers to this system. Instead of talking about the root chakra, I might refer to the "body and everyday physical needs." Rather than saying the "third eye chakra" and talking about intuition, I talk about insight and thought. These words can be understood by all without the umbrella of the chakra system.

The beauty of the ancient chakra system is that it can be applied to just about anything in life. Anything we do, think, say, and feel has the ability to shift our chakras and our collective energy field. Many authors have discussed how to heal the chakras through various means, such as verbal or written affirmations, yogic exercises, or visualization. Since my academic and professional background has been focused on nutrition, I soon began to discern a correlation between food, eating, and chakras. From this perspective, I created a series of classes and workshops called *Nutrition for the Soul* to describe this multidimensional, triangular relationship in an experiential way. These classes prompted me to create the book *Chakra Foods for Optimum*

Health: A Guide to the Foods that can Improve Your Energy, Inspire Creative Changes, Open Your Heart, and Heal Body, Mind, and Spirit in order to take these concepts to a larger audience. While cravings for foods could explain chakra imbalances and eating certain foods could help to correct these imbalances, it seemed that there could be other ways to support the vibration imparted by the foods eaten and how they were eaten. Since I had used dietary supplements extensively in clinical practice, I soon connected the dots and realized that vitamins, minerals, and herbs could be part of that support system. After all, there is a natural connection between food and supplements, as healthy eating patterns often include supplementation. At that point, *Quantum Supplements* was born.

This book will provide you with a hands-on, easy-read, no-nonsense approach to working with your chakras through taking dietary supplements. Please note that this book gives some general guidance on supplements and their relationship to the chakras. With this in mind, I would strongly advise you to work with a healthcare professional to find a supplement regimen tailored to your physical and spiritual needs. *Supplements are not magic bullets.* They provide the space for you to make a shift into the direction of healing. If you start taking supplements, but don't change your life, you will not consistently see the results you are looking for long term. *Therefore, dietary supplements are best used in conjunction with a fully fleshed out healing regimen consisting of a whole-foods way of eating, adequate physical movement, positive thinking and actions, sufficient sleep, and stress management techniques.*

HOW TO USE THIS BOOK

This book is best employed while working with a qualified healthcare professional who is versed in knowledge of the human body and is also open to working with the more subtle layers (for example, emotions, thoughts, spiritual aspects) of the being. You can use the book as a guide, allowing your physical symptoms to usher you to the chapter that serves you at the particular time you need it. If you have a specific body issue that requires attention, check the tables (found in Chapter 2 and in Appendix B) displaying the physiological correlates of the chakras so you will know how to find your way to the chapter containing the information you need.

Let's say that you have been getting frequent colds and would like to know how to bolster your immune system. By checking the chart, you will see that the immune system relates to the root chakra. You would then turn to the chapter on the root chakra for examples of supplemental nutrients or botanicals that could assist you in supporting your immune system. There may be several options, together with recommended daily doses, side effects, and interactions with supplements and drugs. As part of the supplementation strategy, you may also see suggestions listed in that section as to the personal growth or spiritual issues connected to the immune system. For instance, perhaps you need to focus on strengthening your personal boundaries or your ability to say no in situations where it is warranted. This information is not to be ignored. What most people overlook is the deep unfolding process of healing that dietary supplementation can bring forth—instead, they just want the 'quick fix' approach. Rather, the key to optimal health is to embrace the shift that dietary supplements may reveal to you in the direction of healing, and to use this opportunity to fuel positive changes in your life so that you can heal from your symptoms or disease. Foods, eating, and dietary supplements lay the groundwork, but the transformative work still needs to be done by you on other levels (emotional, intellectual, spiritual, etc.).

This book may be employed as a reference manual, or it can be read straight through for a more comprehensive understanding of the finer vibrations of supplements and how they heal the chakras. You will find that several vitamins, minerals, and botanicals will influence more than one chakra. An explanation of a particular supplement is provided in the chapter of the chakra where it has the most effect and includes the following:

- **Description/Sources**: A short detailed definition including what foods it is found in
- **Functions**: How this supplement works in the body
- **Intake**: Who should take this supplement

- **Deficiency**: Symptoms that occur when levels in the body are too low
- **Overuse**: Side effects of high levels in the body
- **Interactions**: How this supplement can interfere with or stimulate the absorption or activity of other supplements and drugs, or how drugs and other supplements can interfere with the absorption or activity of the supplement
- **Relationship to Chakras**: How the supplement affects the subtle energy

If more than one chakra is impacted, that supplement will also be mentioned in the chapter that corresponds to that chakra, with specific instruction as to how it resonates with that particular chakra. For example, vitamin B6 impacts several chakras, but the solar plexus is its primary target since it is required for carbohydrate metabolism. In the chapter on the solar plexus, you will find a detailed explanation of vitamin B6. However, vitamin B6 is also briefly listed under other chakras like the sacral chakra for its role in reducing PMS symptoms and the third eye chakra because it is needed to make neurotransmitters in the brain.

CHAPTER I

INTRODUCTION TO
DIETARY SUPPLEMENTS

Health is a state of complete physical, mental and social
well-being, and not merely the absence of disease or infirmity.
WORLD HEALTH ORGANIZATION, 1948

Today, the average human body confronts an array of modern-day assaults: a nutrient-poor, calorie-rich diet; excessive alcohol consumption; little to no exercise; exposure to environmental toxins like cigarette smoke and pollution, and perhaps significant emotional turmoil, negative thinking, and stress. No wonder we often emerge from the daily battle feeling utterly fatigued, lifeless, and on the verge of breakdown. The body might respond to the injuries by putting on extra weight to protect itself. In the small sliver of time available before significant health issues and eventually a full-blown disease arise, rapid, quick-fix solutions are sought to try to "stop the bleeding."

In the midst of the whirlwind of stress on the body, the spirit attempts to make several cries to the body—"Eat more vegetables," "Get more exercise"—but is not heard. Instead, the body, like a horse with blinders on, fixates on survival in an attempt to get through another day. The spirit's continued urgent pleas to the body remain ignored. The cumulative result of these simultaneous events is a person without passion and purpose for living, who might appear to be moving very mechanically through life, without heart. For example, Jim was in this situation, with his day-to-day life saturated in one challenge after another, including struggling with his income, keeping a job in a tough economy, and tackling some persistent, deep-seated issues with his father. At times, he wanted to give up on everything. A blanket of depression covered him for several weeks. He admitted to himself that he intuitively felt that he needed to be working with plants, but he did not make the effort. When he finally gave in to volunteering at the local greenhouse, he began shifting his life gradually, yet very profoundly. He ended up coming to peace with his family issues and securing a steady position at the community college teaching botany. All of his stresses fell to the background, and he began losing weight and feeling energized.

Body and spirit desire to be unified. The ability to achieve body-spirit wellness rests in the presence of harmony in our lives—with ourselves, others, and the environment. Our highest choice is to be vibrant, healthy, inspired, and full of bountiful energy to give to the thoughts, actions, and emotions that feed our bodies and spirits in the best way. My experience and observations suggest that there are many paths to finding this freedom; one of them is through the vehicle of nourishment. It may not be everyone's path, but those of you who are drawn to using foods and dietary supplements may find it a particularly appealing approach.

As human beings, we need external substances such as food and water to keep us functioning optimally—the bare basics of calories for energy and water to keep hydrated are mere starting points. Under times of stress, when the body is running on overdrive and depleting all of its basic fuel, we may require specific nutrients over and above what we normally take in to give the cells the necessary raw materials they require to harness sufficient energy and remove accumulated waste products. Vitamin C is one of those nutrients that the body uses up quickly during bouts of stress. If we are too low on vitamin C, we leave ourselves open to infection and possibly getting a cold or the flu. On the other hand, eating more citrus fruits or taking a vitamin C supplement during these times protects us from the effects of stress.

Extra, specific supplements enable the physical body to cope with everyday events in ways it otherwise couldn't. When the physical body can flow freely and confidently with the sense of being in control of its surroundings, it has more energy to give to other, "higher" or more spiritual aspects of living. In other words, when our survival needs are taken care of, we are more likely to have the inclination to examine less tangible aspects of our lives like connecting with our life purpose.

Far more than providing just fuel for the physical body, foods and nutritional supplements feed all aspects of us—our flesh, emotions, ego, heart, voice, intuition, and spirit. They do so through their obvious physical qualities like providing calories for energy or minerals for keeping our bones strong. They also contribute in the form of their inherent nonphysical properties: how they were grown, their color and consistency, and how they were prepared and served. Take an example of a chicken egg—you can imagine that eating an egg is an efficient means to get complete protein and energy for the physical body, but its value doesn't end there. If it was produced on a farm where the farmer took good care of the chickens by letting them roam within a spacious area and fed them quality feed, this egg will impart the cumulative, positive effects of the care of the farmer and the healthy, happy life of the chicken that produced the egg. An egg from a well-cared-for chicken may even have different nutrients; it may taste better or even look more robust compared with an egg from a stressed chicken. All around, you would feel good eating it—spanning from your body to your other nonphysical layers. You might even embody the feeling of care and feel its subtle effects in your heart.

Our being, whether physical or nonphysical, collects memories of experiences, words, thoughts, emotions, and actions, which is why those seemingly subtle aspects about how the chicken egg developed are magnified within our being. Quantum physics tells us that every life form carries a vibration, an energetic signature, beyond that of its physical constituents, but definitely connected to its physical parts. In fact, the physical form may be a direct manifestation of all the indirect influences and forces that went into the making of it, just like was described with the chicken egg. It is this subtle vibration that harmonizes with the ethereal, invisible aspects of our being—our subtle, energetic anatomy.

Essentially everything we do, whether we eat certain foods like broccoli or donuts, or take fish oil supplements or eat candy, carries a vibration that will either add to or subtract from the cumulative resonance of the spirit. Eating candy may give us an initial burst of energy from the sugar, but over the long term, and with repeated use, it sets us up to be physically fatigued and drained. The reason for the eventual fatigue is that we put our hormones, especially insulin, on a rollercoaster ride every time we eat too much refined sugar in a repeated fashion. Once in awhile, our bodies may be able to accommodate a sugar rush, but with constant use, our metabolism will have a difficult time riding the waves of chaos sugar creates in the body. Because of these internal imbalances, our energy will be tied up in trying to remedy our body and bring us back into balance. It will have few resources left to invest in the more meaningful, spiritual aspects of our lives. And back we will go to moving through the motions of life rather than fueling it well so that we are glowing, radiant, and full of purpose. *The bottom line is this: eat the energy that you want to become.*

Dietary supplements are unique since they contain higher concentrations of nutrients that we may not normally find in foods. Ingesting them is an efficient way for getting what we need quickly, without the body having to extract the nutrient from the food matrix through the process of digestion.

Let's suppose that we need more minerals like calcium to strengthen our bones or iron for making blood. Yes, we could get these minerals by eating lots of animal foods rich in calcium and iron, but we would have to eat an awful lot of food to get the amount we need, especially if we are seriously depleted or have special needs, like someone with osteoporosis who needs a significant amount of additional calcium or an individual with anemia who needs to replenish their supply of iron. Also, digesting all that food would take a lot of energy. (Animal foods can be especially time consuming and energy intensive for the body to break down and assimilate.)

The food matrix is complex, so, along with essential minerals, we are often ingesting other nutrients from foods that can interfere with the action or digestion of these minerals. But a mineral supplement could cut right to the chase, supplying us with what we need with little to no investment on our part or without the interference of other food constituents that may get in the way.

Now imagine that the person who needs these minerals is a vegetarian. Indeed, they could eat plant foods to get what they needed, but minerals are present in the fabric of plant foods differently from that of animal foods. In plant foods, they are bound to other substances that make it difficult for them to be absorbed unless the foods are cooked well, or, as in the case of iron, have some type of acid applied to it. (For example, lemon juice liberates the iron in spinach leaves to make it available to be absorbed by the body.)

Not only is the matrix of plant foods different, but the quantity of minerals also tends to be lower in plant foods. I'm not implying that vegetarians can't be healthy, only that if we choose to limit our diet to certain foods, we have to be all the more diligent about what we are taking in. And that's why dietary supplements can be so useful. They supply what is needed in a streamlined manner—in a tablet, capsule, powder, or liquid. Using natural supplements along with a sufficient dietary regimen and a healthy lifestyle can produce a great synergy for healing.

I would like to emphasize that dietary supplements are not a quick fix for chronic, deep-rooted issues. They are also not replacements for a healthy diet. They are best used in collaboration with other approaches. Many health issues are best tackled from multiple angles, with foods and supplements not only helping to address body ailments but having an impact on the more subtle aspects of our being like emotions and feeling balanced. Other tactics, like counseling, therapy, journaling, and creative expression, may dive into the depths of the problem straight on. Employing a variety of techniques is often the most successful for healing. This book looks at the role of dietary supplements in the healing process, as one important prong of a multi-pronged approach.

TIPS ON PURCHASING AND STORING SUPPLEMENTS

In order for a dietary supplement to have the intended healing effect, you must give care to exactly what you purchase and how you store it. In addition, while you may find a wide variety of supplement products, including capsules, creams, granules, jellies, liquids, powders, and wafers, at health-food stores, supermarkets, and pharmacies, not all of them are equal when it comes to quality. In fact, a less expensive supplement may be more costly to your health!

The contents of some supplements are also questionable: there can be discrepancies in dose, either too much or too little; and sometimes products are contaminated with substances not intended for the final product. For best results, **always purchase your natural products from a reputable source, preferably a healthcare professional**.

In addition, supplements are only effective to the degree their potency is preserved. Once you purchase your supplements, **protect their potency by storing them in the optimal manner**. Typically, although not always, the way you find supplements in the grocery store is a good indicator of how they need to be kept. For example, probiotics (healthy bacteria for the gut) are usually refrigerated at the store to keep the bacteria alive. You will want to keep them refrigerated when you get them home. B vitamins degrade rapidly in the presence of heat, light, and oxygen, so they are (or should be) kept in a cool, dark place. A food supplement like ground flaxseed meal contains fat that can go rancid if it is not sealed properly to prevent the entry of oxygen. In addition to keeping a tight seal, you might want to refrigerate it to minimize the chances of rancidity.

Guidance on how to keep the supplement is sometimes listed on its label. But if it isn't, you can ask your healthcare professional or read literature on that supplement.

On the product, you will also find an expiration date. **Do not use supplements that are older than their expiration date, as you may not receive their full benefit.** In some cases, they could break down into other compounds that are not necessarily good for the body. For instance, fish oils that are kept too long or are left to degrade may develop a fishy odor, which indicates that they have become rancid.

You will also have to use some common sense when it comes to evaluating the appearance of the supplement. If you are used to a supplement appearing in a certain way—let's say it's a white tablet—and then you notice that the same pills from the same bottle are starting to look a little yellow or developing small specks, that's a good indication that they have changed in some way and you should discontinue use, regardless of the expiration date.

MACRONUTRIENTS

The word *macronutrients* designates nutrients we need to eat in relatively large ("macro") quantities, usually in gram amounts. They include the nutrient trio: carbohydrates, fats, and proteins. There may be times we need special forms of these macronutrients, like a powdered fiber (non-digestible carbohydrate) supplement to support the movement of the gut or a fish-oil capsule to give us the right proportion of essential fats. Macronutrients are used for energy in the body as each of them supplies calories, but they are also involved in maintaining structural and physiological aspects. For example, not only are fats a rich source of energy, but their presence in the cell membrane (the outer wall of a cell) will determine how well that cell will let nutrients and waste products in and out. With a diet too low in unsaturated fats (fats that are fluid at room temperature, like vegetable oils), transport of substances in and out of the cell may be less rapid and the way the cell communicates inside its walls could dramatically change. For example, if your brain does not have sufficient levels of unsaturated fats (particularly the type referred to as "omega-3" fats), it can experience changes in how neurotransmitters flow between nerve cells. In the end, your behavior can even be affected. Insufficient unsaturated omega-3 fats have been associated with mood changes like depression.

The ratio between the three macronutrients is commonly most touted. Active debate in the nutrition community continues on the ideal proportion of carbohydrate, fat, and protein in relation to another—you might be aware of this because these ideas trickle toward consumer awareness in the form of books and radio or TV shows with experts talking about whether the 'ideal' diet should be "low-fat," "low-carbohydrate," or "high-protein," to name a few of the commonly tossed-around diet labels.

PROTEIN

The foundation of the body—the muscle, skin, bones, and immune system—relies on the solid, durable structure of protein. Protein is a highly organized macronutrient that can be disassembled into its amino acid building blocks and used for the layers of muscle, for antibodies that protect the body from outside invaders, and for interlacing circuits of hormones and enzymes. The body would be jelly without protein. Protein allows us to have a structure and the ability to be stable, yet in motion.

There are about twenty essential amino acids that must be eaten in the diet. The body can also make a variety of (nonessential) amino acids. Various types of supplement protein powders are available: soy, whey, rice, pea, and hemp are some of the popular ones. Individuals with allergies to these sources should avoid using them. Soy and dairy are common allergens, which make rice, pea, and hemp viable alternatives. Probably the biggest users of protein powders are people who are interested in bulking up their muscle; however, these powders can be valuable to people who have difficulty keeping on weight (for example, in cancer patients or in those with eating disorders), who want a quality source of protein because they may be missing it in their diet (for example, vegans), or for aging adults when there is a decline in muscle mass. Note: Individuals with kidney disorders should consult with their healthcare professional on the amount of protein they need since too much protein can be taxing for the kidneys.

FAT

Fat is an underestimated, much maligned macronutrient. Unfortunately, the food industry has encouraged some degree of fat phobia by introducing a plethora of "fat-free" products in the 1990s, and health opinion leaders have been chanting the low-fat mantra for several years. As a result, people are skeptical about eating this essential nutrient.

Fat is unique among the macronutrients in that it is the most concentrated source of energy (one gram of fat yields nine calories versus the four calories each from carbohydrates and protein), which is likely the root of its bad reputation. Fat pervades the body: every cell in the body needs a membrane made of fat, and most of our brain tissue (estimates are as high as sixty percent) is fat.

Within the fat nutrient group are **saturated fats** (generally animal-based fats, except tropical oils, like coconut and palm oils) and **unsaturated fats** (typically plant-based fats). The body cannot make certain unsaturated fats (omega-6 and omega-3 fats), so they have been called essential fats, meaning that we *must* eat them. If we don't eat enough of these fats relative to other dietary fats, our vision worsens, our skin becomes rough, our hair can fall out, and our nails fray.

Due to their high quantity in the brain, these fats are also important for behavior. We can't concentrate or feel good without them. Supplemental forms of essential fats include liquid or soft gels containing fish oils (high in omega-3 fats called eicosapentaenoic acid, or EPA, and docosahexaenoic acid, DHA), flaxseed oil, borage-seed oil, and evening primrose oil.

CARBOHYDRATE

The majority of what most people eat (usually fifty to sixty percent of calories) is carbohydrate, a macronutrient used primarily for energy (glucose). Carbohydrates are divided into two categories: simple and complex. **Simple carbohydrates** are very sweet because they are composed of only one or two units of sugar like sucrose (white table sugar), fructose (fruit sugar), and lactose (milk sugar), so they are easy to absorb. **Complex carbohydrates** are longer chains of sugars that typically aren't as sweet because they need to first be broken down into smaller units; some of them (fibers) cannot be fully digested and absorbed, while others (starches) can.

Since carbohydrates, for the most part, readily break down into the simple fuel the body needs, there is a tendency for people to use them to feel energized. One of the best strategies for maintaining energy throughout the day is to ensure that your blood-sugar levels stay constant by eating sufficient amounts of *complex* carbohydrates, or foods/supplements high in fiber. Ideally, it is favorable to eat high-fiber foods like legumes (good examples include lentils, black beans, edamame), vegetables, whole grains (think brown rice instead of white rice!), and some fruits regularly throughout the day. However, there are some individuals who may feel that they need more fiber, whether due to issues they may have with their gut, blood sugar or cholesterol control, or with their bowel movements. For these and perhaps other reasons, it may make sense to use a concentrated fiber supplement (for example, psyllium, flaxseed meal, inulin). It is important to remember, however, to drink adequate water when taking fiber supplements. If you are not used to taking fiber, make sure that you start slow and ramp up to the recommended dose over the course of several days. Without taking these precautions, you may be subject to effects like gastrointestinal bloating, gas, and constipation.

If we are not getting enough complex carbohydrates and eating too many simple ones, we are apt to deplete our energy reserves quickly. Simple carbohydrates like those found in table sugar or fruit juice are rescuer nutrients—like mini life preservers, they come into the body and keep it afloat with a quick burst of energy. The problem is that we can't live our entire lives in short, intense, and repeated energy bursts. Instead, we need long-term, sustained energy to live fully. Fortunately, there is a way to harness and direct our energy with the help of carbohydrates without feeling stressed or depleted. Making the switch from a diet heavy in simple sugars to one that is primarily complex carbohydrates can put us on the path to successfully being able to wield our inner reserves. Once we make this transition, we will encounter less intense cravings for carbohydrates, whether in the form of cookies, pastries, candies, bread, or pasta.

Note that just because dietary supplements have an aura of health doesn't mean that they are perfect in every way. There are some, typically those in liquid or powder form (less in the form of a tablet or soft gel), that may contain significant sources of sugar. A popular one to pay attention to is liquid multi-vitamins, which are often loaded with sugar to mask the off taste of vitamins and minerals. Even children's chewable multivitamins have sugar to make them taste good, supplying another source of sugar in the typically already-high-sugar diet of kids.

Here are some hidden names of sugar to be on the lookout for: **sucrose, high-fructose corn syrup, evaporated cane juice** (commonly found in "healthy" products), **honey, raw sugar, turbinado sugar, brown rice**

syrup, brown sugar, dextrose, corn syrup, maltose. Artificial sweeteners have questionable effects because they are not "natural." Although there have been studies to show they are safe in animals, I do not believe that significant research has been done to support their use in humans. We simply do not know what the potential consequences are for consuming these artificial sweeteners over a lifetime.

There have been a plethora of anecdotes from people claiming to experience side effects like headaches, skin rashes, nausea, or behavior changes like not being able to concentrate and feeling more agitated. I have observed that people who consistently eat artificial sweeteners tend to be prone to more sugar cravings. Because of all the unknowns of how these synthetic ingredients can affect your health, I would recommend avoiding or limiting your intake of all of them: aspartame, Equal®, NutraSweet®, sucralose (Splenda®), and acesulfame potassium. See how much better you feel when you omit them!

MICRONUTRIENTS

Micronutrients are the opposite of macronutrients: they are required in relatively small (micro) amounts compared with the macronutrients. Instead of grams, only 1/1000th of a gram (known as a microgram) of micronutrients is required to meet our bodily needs. Vitamins and minerals fall into this category of nutrients. They can serve as the helpers for the macronutrients and as catalysts for a number of processes. For example, protein provides amino acids like tryptophan, which can be transformed into the neurotransmitter serotonin if vitamin B6 is present in adequate quantities. Similarly, zinc is needed for certain enzymes to convert small-chain essential fats into long-chain fats needed for the brain and eyes.

Historically, vitamin and mineral deficiencies tended to be more common under times of stress, war, or impoverishment. Ironically, even though nowadays in the Western world people eat plenty of food, they are starving for adequate amounts of quality nutrients, particularly micronutrients—indeed, we are paradoxically overfed and undernourished. The U.S. Food and Drug Administration (FDA) has established recommendations for intakes of micronutrients to prevent deficiencies, and these recommendations are tailored for a person's gender and age. Bear in mind that these recommendations do not take into account those who have special needs, such as those on limited diets, on prescription medications, or who smoke or drink alcohol.

Supplements containing vitamins and minerals are easy to locate in a number of stores. They can come in the form of a single ingredient, like calcium tablets with nothing else added, or a nutrient at a high dose, as in a high-potency vitamin C tablet, or as a combination of nutrients, such as calcium, magnesium, and vitamin D for bone health. It is important to recognize that high doses of a single vitamin or mineral may offset levels of another vitamin or mineral and could potentially create an imbalance or relative deficiency. For example, taking too much supplementary zinc can offset copper levels in the body. Along similar lines, some micronutrients work better as a team, such as the family of B vitamins, which act together in the process of extracting energy from macronutrients like carbohydrates.

VITAMINS

Vitamins are required in small amounts to assist overall body processes, like helping the body to digest and metabolize macronutrients. Vitamins are divided into two classes: **fat soluble** and **water soluble.** For the most part, in order for the body to optimally take in fat-soluble vitamins, the vitamins need to be accompanied by a source of fat. So, if you are taking a vitamin E supplement, you would improve its absorption if you took it with a meal containing even a small amount of fat, like a salad with some olive oil dressing. Due to their ability to sink into the fat tissue after ingestion, fat-soluble vitamins are retained in the body for a longer period of time compared with water-soluble vitamins. Fat-soluble vitamins include the following:

- **Vitamin A** (ready-made vitamin A is known as retinol; carotenoids like beta-carotene convert to retinol in the body once ingested)
- **Vitamin D** (plant-derived, vitamin D2 [ergocalciferol], or the form commonly found in animal foods, vitamin D3 [cholecalciferol])
- **Vitamin E** (refers to a whole family of eight compounds, [alpha-, beta-, gamma-, and delta-tocopherol and alpha-, beta-, gamma-, and

delta-tocotrienol] but dietary recommendations focus on alpha-to-copherol, which comes in natural [d-alpha-tocopherol] and synthetic [dl-alpha-tocopherol] forms).

- **Vitamin K** (common supplement forms include vitamin K1 [phylloquinone], vitamin K2 [menaquinone])

On the other hand, water-soluble vitamins are absorbed readily, without fat, but also leave the body quickly through conduits of water like sweat and urine. These vitamins include the **B vitamins** (thiamin [vitamin B1], riboflavin [vitamin B2], niacin [vitamin B3], pantothenic acid [vitamin B5], pyridoxine [vitamin B6], folic acid [vitamin B9], cyanocobalamin [vitamin B12]) and **vitamin C** (ascorbic acid).

MINERALS

Minerals are similar to vitamins in that only minute amounts are needed. Their roles in the body include: maintenance of body pH (the amount of acidity and alkalinity in body compartments, which is very tightly controlled), the formation of bone and blood, nervous system function, muscular contraction and release, and normal enzyme activity.

There is a natural division among the minerals: we require some of them, such as calcium, magnesium, sodium, potassium, and phosphorus, in larger amounts (several hundred milligrams, or even slightly more than a gram), whereas we only require tiny, trace amounts of others, like chromium, copper, iodine, iron, manganese, selenium, and zinc. Vitamins and minerals can both be obtained from foods; however, the difference with minerals is that they usually come from within the earth's crust. Plants take in these minerals from the soil, and the minerals are ultimately eaten by humans or by animals.

HERBS

Herbs have been used since ancient times to cure a host of diseases. Available scientific research suggests that the inner workings of plants may be more complex than those of human beings. They are able to manufacture hundreds of compounds that help them survive in harsh environments, and these compounds have been proposed to be beneficial to the health of humans. Some constituents within a plant may be tied to its healing qualities, such as hypericin in St. John's wort for depression, or silymarin in milk thistle for liver disorders. You will notice that herbal dietary supplements are typically standardized to a certain percentage or amount of a particular compound that has known effects. In some cases, if you don't see this information on the label, you won't know how much of the active compounds you are taking, and, as a result, you could be getting a supplement that may not have the health benefit it is intended to have.

Many of us believe that since herbs have healing properties and are "natural," they can be used indiscriminately. Let me caution you that this is *not* the case. Herbs are very potent substances and can deliver health benefits. In fact, several drugs are derived from plants. **We must use herbs wisely and exercise caution when taking them, the same as we do when we use pharmaceuticals.**

There are many methods of preparation to use herbs internally, in supplement form. Here are a few common ways:

- **Decoctions:** The bark, berry, root, or seed of a plant is boiled to extract certain compounds; it may also be prepared as a tea.
- **Extracts:** Herbs are pressed mechanically and then soaked in water or alcohol. The liquid they were soaked in is then allowed to evaporate. Extracts can also be made by applying heat to the plant matter.
- **Powders:** An herb is ground into a powder, and then the powder is delivered in a capsule or tablet.
- **Tinctures:** An herb is preserved in liquid. The liquid is usually alcohol, but may also be a nonalcohol form, like glycerin.

CHAPTER 2

WHAT ARE CHAKRAS?

*A bodily disease, which we look upon as whole
and entire within itself, may, after all, be but a
symptom of some ailment in the spiritual part.*
NATHANIEL HAWTHORNE

When it comes to the human body, there is much more than meets the eye. Ancient traditions embraced the concept of the person being an interwoven matrix of body, emotions, thoughts, and spirit. We can visualize ourselves as having layers like an onion, one layer tightly nestled on top of the next. The physical layer is what you see when you first meet someone. You see the color of their eyes, their skin, the texture of their hair, the size of their body, and their clothing. When they speak, you may start to formulate some idea about their emotional and mental state. You may start thinking to yourself, "How smart they are! And they seem so happy."

Aside from what we see and assess about people or situations using our five senses, there are more subtle parts of us that add to our analysis. On a less obvious level, each person encompasses the accumulation of all of his likes, dislikes, fears, family issues, phobias, hang-ups about money and relationships, and the culmination of his upbringing, as well as his ability to create and show emotion, be powerful and loving, to communicate effectively, to listen to his intuition, and to connect with Divine guidance. Those multilayered parts of us are wrapped into the fabric of our being and, in a consolidated form, they become a focal point for how we live. We may not be showing them outright, but they collectively make up what we can refer to as our **energy field**, or the nonphysical, bubble-like structure around us that carries the essence of who we are. Some people have expansive energy fields. They walk into a room, and you feel them perhaps before you see them. With others, you may not know they are there until you bump into them. And then there may be circumstances when you are around someone and you start feeling drained, like their energy field has blanketed you.

If we zoom into the anatomy of a person's energy field, we see it is the culmination of many energy threads, and we can dissect the spectrum of different vibrations—these are called *chakras* or *wheels* in Sanskrit, also referred to as "energy centers" throughout this text, all of which correlate to important life issues. "Chakra" is not a new word. Its roots run deep into ancient East Indian texts that are thousands of years old. One way to envision chakras is like invisible doorways for energy to enter and exit our subtle body. Like a revolving door, each chakra lets in energy from the outside and removes it from the inside. There may be times the door opens wide one way but not the other, creating an imbalanced flow of energy, such as when we find ourselves taking care of others more than ensuring that our own basic needs are met. Other times, that door may be whipping open and closed so quickly that the energy in your body may feel overwhelming—this sensation may appear in the body as any number of physical manifestations, such as feeling butterflies in the stomach, the head spinning, the heart racing, and even the classic fight or flight response when we are afraid.

Chakras are positioned in the subtle body and correlate to physical organs. Another way to think about the chakras is like pearls on a necklace, hanging down your spine at the levels of specific endocrine glands. Symbolically, chakras represent a variety of aspects of our being—how we survive, feel, energize, love, speak, intuit, and connect. As we dive within the subtle body landscape, let's approach it from a symbolic perspective. Imagine that the human being has several layers, and in the chakra system, there are seven main ones.

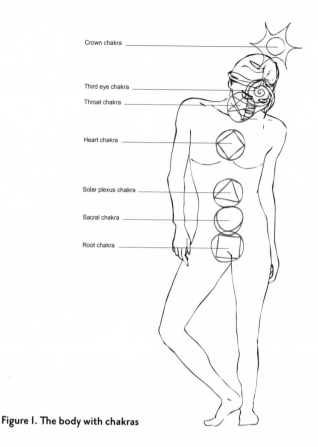

Crown chakra

Third eye chakra

Throat chakra

Heart chakra

Solar plexus chakra

Sacral chakra

Root chakra

Figure I. The body with chakras

The first one is the obvious physical body—flesh and bones. Our physical body connects us symbolically to the issue of survival in the physical world: it allows us to eat, sleep, breathe, and drink. Think of the needs of infants—they need to feel safe, that they can trust, and that they are connected to a family that will provide shelter and food for them. If they didn't have these things, they could not survive. This aspect of our survival stays locked within the vibration of who we are throughout our lives.

You can imagine that if we don't trust or feel safe, we may have some issues with survival, and the opposite is also true. I have seen this with people's eating behaviors, especially in individuals who grew up in poverty. When people do not trust that there will be "enough" for them to survive, they tend to overeat. Conversely, when people do not feel that they have a right to exist, perhaps due to low self-esteem or feeling suicidal, they may tend to forget about eating. They may lose weight and even develop eating disorders.

A person who has an imbalance in her "survival center" doesn't have this energy vibration to a significant degree and may seem like she is "not in her body" by appearing absent-minded, fatigued, or excessively fearful. Sometimes this is referred to as "being ungrounded." The absent-minded professor is a classic example of someone who is so fixated on intellectual concerns that he neglects the needs of the body, like eating or getting enough sleep. A woman who is fearful and worried about survival, whether she is unable to make enough money to support her basic needs or feels her ability to make money is threatened through a potential layoff, may have issues with support not only in the physical world but also in her body. I have seen people in distress like this develop low back pain, knee pain, and sciatica, as their bodies are literally translating the message of not being supported, and so they manifest symptoms of lack of support, particularly in the lower half of the body.

The survival vibrations are instinctual. In ancient traditions, the central point, or hub, of the part of us that resonates with the purely physical aspects of our being and yokes us to the earthly venture of surviving on this planet is called the **root chakra, or muladhara** (Sanskrit for "root"). The designated body location of the root chakra begins the point just under the pubic bone in the front of the body, and penetrates through the body to the level of the tailbone, or coccyx, at the base of the spine. Even though its central point is at the level of the tailbone, its energetic influence is directed downwards toward the lower half of the body, into the legs and feet.

Once we are comfortable with feeling grounded in our physical body and the elements that comprise much of our basic survival needs as they relate to the physical world, we are then able to direct our energy up the body to the next energy center, which is the font of raw emotions and creativity. Think of the infant becoming a toddler: screaming, crying, demanding, giggling—the "terrible twos" as they are called. We are now moving past our basic survival needs and into the realm of feeling. As a young child, we find our own inner voice, we begin playing with others, and amplifying our every need. If we take this into the adult life, this part of us translates into our ability to be freely creative, have fun, express how we feel, and develop relationships. To some extent, this is the part of us that psychologists refer to as the "inner child."

There are various ways this aspect manifests when it is out of balance: a workaholic who makes no time for play, a woman who isn't comfortable showing her emotions and so she stuffs them in by eating, the tortured artist type who feels that his feelings and creative expression are misunderstood, a person who has difficulty committing to a relationship or maintaining friendships.

The energetic part of us associated with our ability to be creative, wildly emotional, and full of pleasure is kept in the area between our lower belly (just below the navel) and the sacrum. It is referred to as the **sacral chakra,** or **svadhisthana** (Sanskrit for "one's own abode"). Think of how when you laugh heartily or breathe deeply—your lower gut feels relaxed and free of tension. Whereas the root chakra is symbolically associated with our ability to feel grounded and secure in our bodies, the sacral chakra has been likened to the aspect of us that embodies the water element through its flowing, yet still, abysmal depth; our expanse of emotion; and our ability to dive into the unconscious. When we are in touch with our lower gut and its energetic resonance, we dance to the music of our raw creativity, our unruly emotions, and our love of companionship. These parts of us ripple through our gut and undulate into finer expression with the help of the heart (love and passion) and throat (voice and authenticity) chakras. This chakra seeks relationship with another. It propels us out to the world to find connection and synergy. When we are deeply committed to our own sensitivity and creativity, we can be open to sharing this beauty with another, and in this process, create something anew.

Swimming upwards from the low belly, we enter our fiery, transformative energy-exchange center. With the vehicle of the body (root chakra) and the ability to emote, create, and form relationships with others (sacral chakra), we now have the tools needed to make our way in the world, and to *exchange the energy* of our self with the energy of society. If we can symbolically position this stage of our development, it would be at the ages of five to seven years old, when we are forming and solidifying our identity.

It has been said that who we were at this young age sets the stage for who we are to become as adults. We begin to have strong views, develop opinions, and have a sense of self as separate from the whole. Individuals with imbalances in this center often has issues around self-worth. For example, they are often the ones who can never have enough material possessions to give them a sense of worth. They continue to collect and hoard but ultimately receive no gratification in return. An overachiever seeks to find fulfillment through her accomplishments rather than who she is from within. Sometimes the most egocentric person is masking low feelings of self-worth; in other words, all that grandiosity is not who they really are. When it comes to foods and eating, these individuals are hungry for internal fulfillment and confidence, and may use external sources like foods and overeating in an attempt to fill this need.

The part of us that filters societal information and allows us to distill our own opinions, beliefs, and identity is held in the upper abdominal area and is known as the **solar plexus chakra,** or **manipura** (Sanskrit for "city of jewels"). The middle of the torso is the energetic home for the essential organs of transformation associated with the solar plexus chakra: the gallbladder, liver, pancreas, small intestines, and stomach. Energy, whether from the purely physical like food or from a charged interaction with a group of people at work, will enter in from the outside and is converted through this conduit into a form that we can process and recognize. In response to taking in the energy, we may even decide to give back energy from this center through movement, activity, and acting from our core.

An example of this exchange might be the simple act of eating a meal. The body sees the food as a vehicle of energy and breaks it down to the degree that it can reap the energy embedded within. As a result of taking in this energy, we may feel more alive, invigorated, and propelled into action. That energy may help us exercise, move through the day, and do our tasks.

The three lower chakras, the root, sacral, and solar plexus centers, form the physical basis of a person. The root chakra could be compared to the bricks of a house, giving a solid structure and foundation. The sacral chakra is like the windows built into the house, allowing us to see to the outside using our senses and our urge to connect with others. And the solar plexus chakra is like the front and back doors, enabling people to enter and for the inhabitants to exit.

From this point on, the chakras become much more ethereal in nature, and they are aligned more closely with the spirit than the body. Although no more significant than the lower three chakras, the upper four chakras have more delicate and finer vibrations than those of the lower chakras. Collectively, the upper chakras encompass the parts of a person that allows them to love, communicate, think, and connect with the Divine. If we continue with the metaphor of the house, they go beyond the house structure and take us into the periphery: into other neighborhoods, cities, countries, and even dimensions.

The journey of the upper chakras begins with the much-cherished **heart chakra,** or **anahata** (Sanskrit for "unstruck" or "unbeaten"). Common expressions such as "living from the heart" or "following your heart" have infiltrated people's lives, as has the ubiquitous heart symbol, which has made its way onto everything from t-shirts and lunchboxes to bumper stickers and greeting cards. The heart chakra is unique because it bridges the physical and the spiritual aspects (sometimes referred to as the "heaven and earth") of a person through love.

Coming from the place of the heart center enables us to smooth any gaps between our body and spirit, and once this connection has been made, we are able to extend it to others by giving and receiving love through sound, song, and embrace. The heart chakra keeps the physical heart and lungs circulating with currents of blood and oxygen. Without the heart chakra and its organs, the body is unable to live on the earth plane of existence.

Working upwards from the heart chakra in the center of the chest is the **throat chakra,** or **vishuddha** (Sanskrit word for "pure wheel"), which oversees the throat, thyroid gland, mouth, ears, and nose. The throat has been likened to a birthing canal for the heart: it is the part of us that is responsible for choices we make, and we express those choices and who we are through the vehicle of the voice. In its highest form, it speaks the language of the heart.

Since there is choice and communication involved in this center, it also has a connection to a more refined form of creativity than that of the sacral chakra. The sacral chakra births raw ideas in a primitive form, and the throat chakra sculpts them according to the wishes of the heart. The throat chakra provides the physical manifestation of vibration through chanting, singing, and spoken words. It is also the point of entry for much of the energy that is exchanged through the solar plexus chakra, since the throat chakra can take in food, liquid, dietary supplements, and sensory input through the mouth, ears, and nose, and give out words in response to what the solar plexus chakra is processing.

All the energy exchange, sensory input, and communication produce thoughts. The activity of the brain falls within the realm of the **third eye chakra,** or **ajna** (Sanskrit word for "command"). Logically formed thoughts, emotional pattern recognition, and the master control center for much of the body's hormones live within this chakra's rapid vibratory rate. Think of the speed of a thought or the blink of an eye; this quick and dynamic energy reflects the resonance of this chakra.

The chakras are largely vessels of transition, places of our invisible, energetic landscape that funnel energy in all forms through the ethers into the flesh, and from the flesh into the ethers. The third eye chakra spins in many directions, gathering and receiving energy like an antenna, from many sources. It may be processing information from the physical plane, or it may be receiving signals from abstract, otherworldly places. So the third eye manages not only thoughts, but also intuitive insight that may be an amalgam of our earthly experiences and universal guidance underlying a Divine plan.

Finally, the **crown chakra,** or **sahasrara** (Sanskrit for "the supreme center of contact with God") sits at the top of the head like a halo. It has the finest, lightest vibration of all the major seven chakras, and it feeds the body with cellular intelligence, universal consciousness, and life force. It represents our direct line to the spiritual part of us, the essence of us that knows no time, boundaries, form, or opposites. When we are in union with this part of ourselves, through prayer or meditation, we remember our true nature and origin and their spiritual roots.

Chakra (Sanskrit Name)	Physical Location	Anatomical and Physiological Association	Connection with Major Life Issues
Root (Muladhara)	Base of spine, perineum	Adrenal glands, bones, DNA, feet, immune system, joints, legs, muscles, prostate gland, rectum, red blood cells, male reproductive organs, skin, tailbone	Feeling safe and able to trust others, meeting physical needs to survive as a human being, belonging to a tribe (family, society), developing structure and boundaries, protecting the self
Sacral (Svadhisthana)	Sacrum, low belly below navel and above pubic bone	Bladder, hips, kidneys, large intestine (colon), ovaries, sacrum, urinary tract, uterus	Relating with another, expressing emotions, engaging in pleasure and play, liberating creativity
Solar Plexus (Manipura)	Middle back, solar plexus region at level of diaphragm	Gallbladder, liver, pancreas, small intestine, stomach	Manifesting personal power in the world, interacting with the external world, harnessing and expending energy
Heart (Anahata)	Upper back, middle chest	Armpits, arms, blood vessels, breasts, hands, heart, lungs, lymphatic system, shoulders, wrists	Expressing love, giving and receiving love, loving the self and others, displaying gratitude, expressing feelings from a place of emotional wisdom
Throat (Vishuddha)	Cervical spine, throat	Cheeks, chin, ears, larynx, lips, mouth, neck, nose, pharynx, thyroid gland, throat, tongue, upper esophagus	Releasing control and accepting one's life path, speaking one's truth, honoring the senses, expressing the self through words
Third Eye (Ajna)	Between eyebrows, on forehead	Brain, eyebrows, eyes, forehead, neurotransmitters, pineal and pituitary glands (which regulate hormone function)	Processing thoughts, dreaming, receiving higher guidance, following one's intuition, being receptive to insight, separating truth from illusion
Crown (Sahasrara)	Top of head	Cellular intelligence, central nervous system	Trusting one's higher self, believing in a power or force greater than oneself, surrendering to a greater power, acknowledging the interconnection of all of life

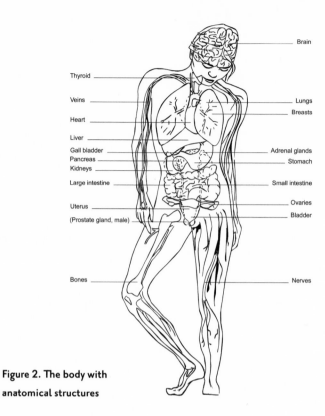

Figure 2. The body with
anatomical structures

CHAPTER 3

THE INTERRELATIONSHIP BETWEEN HERBS, SUPPLEMENTS, AND CHAKRAS

It was not meant that the soul should cultivate the earth,
but that the earth should educate and maintain the soul.
MARGARET FULLER (1810–1850), *Memoirs*

Depending on our life choices, the process of living may dull, dim, or deplete the vivid rainbow of energy we are composed of. Since everything that surrounds us carries an energy signature, it would be reasonable that we could tweak, shift, repair, and restore our rainbow energy with the assistance of external sources. Because we eat every day, one way to change our energy is through foods. Indeed, people can eat specific foods to help heal the chakras.

This concept and its application are described in detail in my previous book, *Chakra Foods for Optimum Health*. However, sometimes food is not enough. We may experience repeated injury and long-term imbalance in the energetic field, resulting from compounded everyday stresses and burdens. To assist in the healing process, some people find that supplementing their healthy eating regimen and lifestyle approach with additional, fine-tuned nutritional or herbal support helps restore and shift their subtle energy to carry a different vibration—ultimately one that supports optimal wellness.

The distilled vibratory essence of foods and plants in supplement form can affect the vibration of the chakras. When ingesting any number of the 29,000 dietary supplements on the market, people are most likely attempting to balance the life issues the chakras represent on a more philosophical and even spiritual level, but perhaps they are not always aware they are doing so. For example, not everyone realizes that high cholesterol and heart issues may be signs of deeper issues within the heart chakra—that is, how love is given and received, and even whether one has difficulty loving oneself. But if you examine the connection beyond the laboratory measurement of cholesterol, the relationship seems to be a logical one. The body-spirit paradigm is not new. Fortunately, it is on the verge of shifting into greater visibility, which may lead to increased awareness of the multilayered reasons for symptoms and, ultimately, enhanced healing.

Based on this model, certain nutrients resonate with one or more chakra centers. Like the healing effects of foods, the healing effects of these potent nutrients are determined by their physical properties (solid, liquid, oil, powder, plant extract), origin, color, and function in the body. Pigments, minerals, vitamins, and plants are all part of the palette of dietary supplements used in the art of healing the chakras. For example, the colorful compound which is available in dietary supplement form, beta-carotene, a well-known orange-red plant pigment that converts in the body to vitamin A, imparts its orange color vibration and protective properties as an antioxidant to serve a deficient sacral chakra. Since its origin is carrots, a root vegetable, beta-carotene also extends its energy to the root chakra.

Minerals, through their contribution to physiological structure and, eventually, to function, stabilize the energy flow to and from chakras. This concept is seen with the mineral supplements zinc and iron, which compose the anatomical matrix governed by the root chakra. (For example, zinc is a component of protein-containing enzymes, and iron composes red blood cells.) Vitamins, either singly or in combination, may orchestrate activities in the chakras. If it weren't for the family of B vitamins working together as a team (referred to as the "B complex"), the solar plexus chakra would not be able to metabolize carbohydrates for energy. And, finally, plant extracts can be taken as a supplement to promote the vibration of healthy chakras; St. John's wort, for instance, can be taken to support healthy mood and third eye chakra activity. Along these same lines, ginkgo extract helps with memory and cognitive function, both of which fall within the realm of the third eye chakra.

MACRONUTRIENTS AND THEIR CONNECTION TO THE CHAKRAS

As discussed earlier in Chapter 2, the lower three chakras, the root, sacral and solar plexus centers, tend to be more connected to the physical body than do the upper four chakras. As a result, the major macronutrients, protein, fat, and carbohydrate, correspond respectively to these chakras:

- **Protein and the root chakra**: Protein provides the basis for the strong support of body tissues that are governed by the root chakra, like muscles, bones, skin, and the immune system. On an energetic (symbolic) level, it gives an individual a sense of stability, safety, and trust by imparting its "building" energy, or ability to form new structures. Real-world example of how this manifests: High-protein diets became a popular trend after the terrorist attack on the Twin Towers in New York City in 2001, possibly in an effort to promote a sense of safety and security in society at large.
- **Fat and the sacral chakra**: Fat is needed in the body for establishing flow, whether flow of menstrual blood, waste through the kidneys and colon, or communication between cells. On an energetic (symbolic) level, it enables us to effectively express creativity, emotions, and the senses. The nature of the fat represents its effects in the body: the more liquid and flowing the fat, the more it contributes to the expression of aspects of the self. Real-world example of how this manifests: Many people, especially women, are fat-phobic and will

not eat dietary fat because they fear it will "make them fat." Although this has been debunked by science, the perception remains. Adding to this observation, I have noticed that women who avoid fat also seem to have difficulty expressing emotions. They tend to become preoccupied with stuffing the emotion down with food rather than letting the emotion come out and be fully expressed.

- **Carbohydrate and the solar plexus chakra**: Carbohydrates, whether sugars or starches, are burned for energy in the body, and this energy is used to fuel activity, including defining who we are through our outward projection of a job or career, accomplishments, or expression of our opinions, desires, and dreams. On an energetic (symbolic) level, it imparts to us the ability to harness our energy and be powerful. Real-world example of how this manifests: In today's society, most people's lives are full of stress. One way that we cope with stress and from being worn out from the exchange of energy that happens repeatedly, consistently throughout the day, is by sinking into sweet foods: the rush from candy, cookies, and soft drinks gets us to the next moment. However, at the end of the day, we feel even more depleted and empty, physically and spiritually.

VITAMINS, MINERALS, AND HERBS AND THEIR CONNECTION TO THE CHAKRAS

On an energetic level, micronutrients support all of the energy centers of the body. Whereas the macronutrients provide the general body structure and connect strongly to the lower chakras (root, sacral, and solar plexus chakras), vitamins and minerals support the body's ability to be animated— to function and be active—by serving as catalysts in a multitude of biochemical reactions. Although they are needed in lesser amounts, their importance to the body is not small.

The fact that vitamins and minerals can work together either synergistically or antagonistically is relevant from an energetic perspective as well:

the circuit of energy centers is interdependent. If a single energy center is deficient in a micronutrient, the effect cascades through to the whole energy circuit. When certain vitamins and minerals are taken together, they may assist more than one chakra at a time.

From an energetic perspective, vitamins are the vital substances that invigorate the human being, allowing it to come to life. Without vitamins, we wouldn't be able to hold the current of life energy within us or to extract it from foodstuffs. Consequently, minerals provide a direct conduit to the healing, grounding energy of the earth and resonate strongly with the root chakra, or the earthy, primarily bodily composition of a human being. An herb carries an energetic vibration that is quite different from the vibrations of macronutrients and micronutrients. Macronutrients have a steady resonance, almost like the consistent beat of the heart. They are parental and guardianlike, shepherding the body into existence and providing sustenance for function. The micronutrients are the energetic helpers of the macronutrients; the two have a strong interrelationship. On the other hand, herbs are in a category all their own. Since they are independent life forms, their energy is more complex and multidimensional than that of the isolated nutrients, making their effects very potent. They can impact all of the energy centers, even simultaneously. Their potency is not unreasonable to fathom considering that the origin of many pharmaceuticals is based on plant compounds.

CHAPTER 4

SUPPLEMENTS FOR GROUNDING AND PROTECTION (ROOT CHAKRA)

It is only by grounding our awareness in the living sensation
of our bodies that the "I Am," our real presence, can awaken.

G.I. GURDJIEFF

CHAKRA DESCRIPTION

The physical world we live in has its roots in a dense, slow-moving vibration. Sometimes it may feel as though we are living in slow motion—we spend our days working long hours, in congested traffic, and our health may not change as quickly as we'd like. The nuts and bolts of our survival are what our root chakra brings to our energy palette. How we live—our shelter, our family, our meals—are all components that take time to create, grow, and experience. Think of the steady, consistent time it takes to go to school for a degree, to save up enough money to buy a house, or to procure a job we enjoy. All of these aspects of everyday living funnel into the energy of the root chakra, and the time it takes for them to come into existence mirrors the methodical, gradual layering process embraced by the steady vibration of this center.

Words associated with the root chakra: *ancestors, being present, blood, body, earth, family/tribe, flesh, grounded, instinct, nature, origins, physical matter, protection, red, safety, security, survival.*

CHAKRA ANATOMY AND PHYSIOLOGY

The root chakra gives us a physical form—starting with DNA, our ancestral life force; the warm river of blood that runs through us; our immune defenses that ward off invaders; and the large framework of our skeleton and muscle tissue. It governs excretion through the rectum and creation in men through the sperm produced by the prostate gland. The outer layer of the skin provides the visible barrier to the external world. Overall, the root chakra gives our being its origin and protects that creation through internal and external defenses.

Root chakra anatomy: Adrenal glands, blood cells (red and white), bones, DNA, feet, immune system, joints, legs, muscle, prostate gland, rectum, reproductive organs (male), skin and tailbone.

HEALTHY INDICATIONS

A person who is comfortable with their physical self (root chakra) is someone who knows they can survive adequately in the world; is comfortable with receiving from or providing support to a family or tribe; is trustworthy and trusts others; accepts himself, especially their physical body and their earthly existence; maintains healthy boundaries; believes they have has a right to exist.

UNHEALTHY INDICATIONS

If you answer yes to a majority of the following questions, your root chakra may need healing:

- *Do you feel out of place within or at war with your family of origin?* People with root chakra imbalances usually have not come to terms with challenging family issues, especially those involving acquiring a home or shelter, making a living, and carrying on family traditions. These individuals often find it difficult to bond with family members in a way that is meaningful and solidifies a feeling of unity and cohesion.
- *Do you constantly feel on guard or that you have to expend much of your internal resources to be safe or to defend yourself?* Spending significant

energy to feel safe, whether constantly being on guard physically by being especially careful about your possessions or even trying to protect yourself emotionally like not getting too close to someone for fear that you will be hurt, may ultimately deplete the energy reserves meant to protect you from physical invaders, like microorganisms, viruses, excess inflammatory compounds, and toxins. Lower internal (immune) defenses may ultimately lead to symptoms of fatigue, frequent cold or flu, or inflammatory or autoimmune conditions.

- *Do you struggle with the idea of life and the process of living?* Individuals with root chakra imbalances find everyday life to be difficult and not worth the effort. They can lack motivation and appear lazy to others, and may enter a deep depression. When root chakra imbalances along these lines exist, the individuals can appear spacey, flighty, or "not all there." In fact, it is almost as if the individual is not in their body. And truly, they are not in their body—or their root chakra—on an energetic level. Without being fully present, we are unable to live life fully and to manifest our dreams.

- *Do you fear having "enough," especially when it comes to food?* Are you preoccupied with your food resources—how much you have at any one time, or how much of your finances you allocate to food? Some of us have had strong messages about lack rather than abundance and guilt instead of gratitude programmed into us even as children (remember hearing, "Kids in Africa are starving so you better eat everything on your plate!"?). These built-in messages make us fearful about our existence. Since the root chakra is about survival, and food is fundamental to our physical functioning, it follows that most food issues can be traced back to the root chakra.

SUPPLEMENTS FOR THE ROOT CHAKRA

Because the root chakra connects with the physical nature of a human being, several supplements are associated with this chakra. Often, our root chakra is the aspect of us that most needs healing, and, fortunately, it is responsive to physical substances like food and supplements.

MACRONUTRIENTS AND MACRONUTRIENT SUPPLEMENTS

Protein

Protein is the main macronutrient associated with the root chakra. It provides the building blocks (amino acids) for the body's gross anatomical structure: bone, muscle, and skin. We obtain most of our protein through our diet when we eat animal-based foods like meat, yogurt, milk, eggs, and cheese, and hearty plant-based foods such as beans and nuts. We can also get protein through high-quality, protein-based supplement powders. Due to its animal origin (which is highly grounding, or brings us back into the present moment, helping us to focus) and ability to support muscle tissue and the immune system, one of the best supplement powders for the root chakra is whey protein; however, other protein powders (rice, soy, or pea protein) are also effective. When you are feeling particularly spaced-out or flighty (which I like to call "ungrounded"), try drinking a shake made in the blender using whey protein powder and red fruits like raspberries or strawberries. (Red is the color that feeds the root chakra.) For individuals who may have difficulty digesting protein, partially degraded proteins, like hydrolyzed whey protein, are an option. All individual amino acids, particularly those that are essential because the body cannot make them (including isoleucine, leucine, lysine, methionine, phenylalanine, threonine, tryptophan, and valine) in a supplement support the function of the root chakra.

When protein digestion is a problem: People with imbalanced root and solar plexus chakras may have difficulty digesting and assimilating protein; this difficulty is indicated by stomach bloating immediately or shortly after eating. As we advance in age, our stomach tends to make less hydrochloric acid, a strong acid produced in the stomach to denature and digest proteins. Without this acid, our ability to digest and take in protein is significantly impaired. Bacteria could cause the undigested food in the stomach to ferment, which results in bloating. A chronic lack of stomach acid coupled with a more permeable ("leaky") gut caused by bacterial overgrowth results in a lack of discrimination as to which molecules get absorbed. This is especially problematic since the absorption of large, undigested proteins may result in a heightened immune response.

For those with low stomach-acid production (a condition referred to as achlorhydria), hydrochloric acid (HCl) supplements are useful. In some cases, they can be beneficial for individuals with food allergies and autoimmune diseases like rheumatoid arthritis. HCl supplements are usually found as betaine HCl; betaine is a carrier for the HCl. An HCl supplement must be taken carefully. For example, it should not be taken if you are taking an NSAID (a nonsteroidal anti-inflammatory drug, such as aspirin or ibuprofen) or corticosteroid (such as prednisone), since the combination may cause severe gastric upset. Betaine HCl, in the form of tablet or capsule, is to be taken midway through a large, protein-containing meal. Various dosage recommendations exist. You can start at the minimum dose (600 milligrams) and see whether you experience less bloating and stomach upset. If you do not, try gradually increasing the dose until your symptoms are relieved. **Taking too much betaine HCl can lead to a sharp heartburn sensation so ensure that you start slowly to be sure that you find the dose that is right for you.**

If you struggle with protein digestion, try examining this on a more symbolic level. Take note of what might be particularly "difficult to digest" in terms of information relating to your family of origin, to your job, or to making ends meet. When we feel overwhelmed by circumstances relating to survival, we may not be able to assimilate external energy effectively in our root chakra. Through its energetic link to the root chakra, the solar plexus chakra, which oversees such digestive organs as the stomach, may be impacted to the extent that the body cannot use energy from the outside (especially protein). The stomach bloats, unable to process the energy it receives, and over time, without adequate protein, the internal protein reserves are mobilized. The end result is the deterioration and wasting away of the anatomical structures and physiological functions of the root chakra (for example, delayed wound healing, hair loss, immune impairment, skin peeling, and muscle breakdown).

Carbohydrate

Insoluble fiber, or the type of chewy fiber that speeds the passage of foods through the digestive tract, helps ensure healthy bowel movements (the root chakra oversees the rectum and excretory functions of the body) and, therefore, the release of toxins. Without enough fiber in our diet, we could develop constipation and hemorrhoids. Dietary supplement powders containing cellulose or bran (for example, wheat bran and rice bran), both insoluble fibers, would be beneficial. It is advised that you take supplemental fiber separate from other supplements (especially minerals) or medications, because the fiber can potentially bind the supplement or drug and make it unavailable for absorption.

Insoluble fiber imparts the root chakra energy of protection since it is typically derived from the outer sheaths, or protective layers, of plants (such as the skin of fruit and the bran layer of grains). Also, insoluble fiber is commonly found in (root) vegetables, one category of foods that nourishes root chakra energy. The characteristics of this fiber—tough, tenacious, indestructible—mirror the grounded nature intended by the root chakra.

VITAMINS

Vitamin A (retinol, carotenoids)

Description and Sources: Fat-soluble vitamin commonly found as preformed vitamin A (retinol) in animal foods such as meat, eggs, and whole milk. Some colorful plant compounds called carotenoids are able to convert to the active form of vitamin A after they have been ingested. Of all the hundreds of carotenoids, beta-carotene, the orange pigment in carrots and other orange fruits and vegetables, has the highest conversion rate to active vitamin A in the body.

Functions: When taken orally, it can improve immune system, skin and mucosal surfaces, cell division and growth, bone development, eye health, and embryonic development, and it may play role in inhibiting cancer development. Also used in topical applications for skin-health benefits (reducing wrinkles, ultraviolet [UV] protection, and wound healing).

Intake: Individuals with long-term fat malabsorption such as in celiac disease or Crohn's disease may be more susceptible to developing vitamin A deficiency. Vegans need to ensure that they get adequate precursor carotenoids by eating copious amounts of fruits and vegetables or by taking a vitamin A supplement. One study showed that vitamin A was one of the nutrients important for preventing cataracts. The Institute of Medicine has commented that beta-carotene supplementation may not be suitable for the general population due to two studies that resulted in greater incidence of cancer in people taking beta-carotene. In one of the studies, the population was smokers. As a result, there are mixed opinions as to whether smokers should take vitamin A.

Deficiency: Decreased immune function, night blindness that can proceed to vision loss if not treated, increased risk of infection.

Overuse: Short-term, high doses (15,000 micrograms, or 50,000 units) can cause nausea, vomiting, headache, spinal pressure, and blurred vision. Taking 30,000 micrograms (100,000 units) or more for long periods of time (months, years) can result in liver toxicity, fatigue, irritability, drastic behavioral changes, nausea, vomiting, and itchy, red skin. Too much vitamin A intake can have a negative effect on bone. Intakes of greater than or equal to 3,000 micrograms (10,000 units) daily have been shown to increase the risk for osteoporosis and hip fractures in postmenopausal women.

Interactions: Use caution when taking vitamin A together with drugs that can negatively impact liver function. Avoid concomitant use with retinoids (vitamin A derivatives such as isotretinoin), tetracycline antibiotics, and with anticoagulant supplements and drugs (for example, warfarin). Advise your healthcare practitioner if you are pregnant, nursing, or if you smoke, before taking vitamin A.

Relationship to Chakras: Primary chakra: root. Secondary chakras: sacral, solar plexus, heart, throat, third eye. Since vitamin A is so integral to the physical body in various ways, it exhibits the greatest resonance with the root chakra more than other chakras. Specifically, it interfaces with the root chakra because it helps regulate immunity and promote skin integrity. However, it is also strongly linked to the throat chakra, because it is needed for maintaining healthy mucous membranes; to the third eye chakra via its ability to promote healthy eyes and night vision; and to the solar plexus chakra, since most of the body's vitamin A is stored in the liver. Carotenoids, which are the colorful pigments in plants, such as the orange pigment beta-carotene, are pre-vitamin A compounds. When they are eaten, they convert to vitamin A in the body. Since these compounds resonate with the sacral and heart chakras, vitamin A is also remotely linked to these energy centers.

Vitamin B5

See chapter on the solar plexus chakra for more details. Because of its role in the functioning of the adrenal gland, vitamin B5 (pantothenic acid) is required under high stress conditions and for those who experience adrenal exhaustion (characterized by fatigue, sleep disturbances, headache, to name a few symptoms). The recommended therapeutic dose for those experiencing chronic stress is 100 to 500 milligrams daily.

Folic Acid

Description and Sources: Folate is a water-soluble vitamin present in a wide variety of foods, including leafy green vegetables (the origin of the word "folate" is "folium," which means "leaf" in Latin), fruits, whole grains, legumes, and some meats. The supplemental form of folate, referred to as folic acid, is found in dietary supplements and processed foods.

Functions: Since this vitamin assists in the formation of red blood cells and white blood cells, it is important for preventing anemia and for maintaining healthy immune function. It is a core nutrient required for healthy cell division and growth. Because of its role in protein metabolism, folic acid, together with vitamins B6 and B12, converts the amino acid homocysteine into nonharmful amino acids in the body. Elevated homocysteine has been shown to be associated with increased incidence of atherosclerosis (blood vessel narrowing due to the build-up of plaque).

Intake: Folate/folic acid intake is important for women who intend to become pregnant, and pregnant women, particularly early in the pregnancy, because it is needed for embryonic and fetal nerve cell development. If inadequate folic acid is available during pregnancy, neural tube defects (deformities in the skull, brain, and spine) in the developing fetus can result. When taken in conjunction with vitamins B6 and B12, it may also be useful in individuals with high levels of homocysteine in their blood. Individuals who have gut malabsorption and liver disease may be particularly vulnerable to low folic acid intakes.

Deficiency: Anemia, fatigue, gastrointestinal upset, sore, red tongue, growth impairment, insomnia, memory problems, paranoia, weakness, birth defects.

Overuse: Relatively low toxicity, but high doses can result in abdominal cramps, diarrhea, rash, altered sleep patterns, and neurological disturbances. Daily doses of 1,000 micrograms should not be exceeded, because too much folate can mask a deficiency of vitamin B12.

Interactions: May interfere with the actions of methotrexate (used for cancer) and with antiseizure drugs—check with a healthcare practitioner before using folic acid supplements if you are on either of these medications. Not to be taken for extended periods if a history of cancer or seizure disorder is present: high supplemental folic acid (not less than 1 milligram) has been associated with increased seizures; folic acid supplementation may theoretically increase cancer occurrence by stimulating cell growth. In case of anemia, do not supplement with folic acid unless your healthcare practitioner determines the type of anemia you have (folic acid can mask anemia due to vitamin B12 deficiency, ultimately leading to nerve damage).

Relationship to Chakras: Primary chakra: root. Secondary chakras: sacral, heart, third eye. Folic acid is key to the functions of the root chakra, since both folic acid and the root chakra are concerned with cell growth and maintaining immune function. In pregnant women, it is especially needed by the sacral chakra for fetal growth and development. Because it helps to reduce homocysteine, it serves as a protector of the blood vessels, which are nurtured by the heart chakra. Finally, folic acid is involved in production of healthy neurotransmitters in the brain, thus assisting the third eye chakra in its role to balance moods.

Vitamin B12 (cyanocobalamin, methylcobalamin)

Description and Sources: A reddish, water-soluble vitamin found in animal foods such as meat, eggs, fish, milk, and shellfish; it can also be manufactured by microorganisms.

Functions: Needed to prevent anemia. Plays a vital role in cell growth, DNA synthesis, and acts as a cofactor for fat and carbohydrate metabolism. Assists in the synthesis of myelin, the fatty sheaths that protect nerves, and hence, influences nerve-cell activity. Together with folic acid and vitamin B6, it regulates homocysteine levels. Required for acetylcholine production in the brain for memory and learning.

Intake: Supplementation is encouraged for vegetarians and for those who have difficulty absorbing nutrients due to stomach or intestinal conditions.

Deficiency: Depression, abnormal gait, fatigue, changes in digestion, dizziness, drowsiness, headaches, pernicious anemia, neurological disorders, skin sensitivity.

Overuse: Typically no toxic effects from high amounts.

Interactions: High doses of folic acid can mask vitamin B12 deficiency. A number of medications, including aspirin, antibiotics, and oral contraceptives, can reduce the absorption or activity of vitamin B12 in the body.

Relationship to Chakras: Primary chakra: root. Secondary chakras: solar plexus, heart, third eye, crown. Vitamin B12 is a core nutrient for the root chakra because of its role in cellular growth and DNA synthesis. Without its contribution, root chakra energy could be left depleted, and the physiological outcome would manifest as anemia. Moving up from the root chakra, vitamin B12 feeds the energy-harnessing task of the solar plexus chakra by playing an assisting role in metabolism. Together with folate and vitamin B6, vitamin B12 works to reduce levels of homocysteine, an unwanted compound that causes stuck energy in the circulation governed by the heart chakra. Finally, the third eye and crown chakras are impacted through vitamin B12's effects on memory and the nervous system. The uniqueness of this vitamin is its ability to provide the full spectrum of energetic resonance, spanning from the grounded energy of the root chakra to the finer vibration of the crown chakra.

Vitamin C (ascorbic acid)

Description and Sources: Sour, water-soluble compound found in fruits and vegetables, especially citrus fruits.

Functions: Most recognized for its antioxidant action (cell protection against free radicals) and ability to enhance the immune system. Also plays part in collagen (protein) synthesis and the metabolism of amino acids, like tyrosine and phenylalanine. Responsible for balancing stress hormones involved in fight-or-flight response, like norepinephrine and cortisol. The adrenal glands (overseen by the root chakra) contain one of the highest concentrations of vitamin C in the body.

Intake: Increased amounts, as much as 600 to 1,000 milligrams per day, have been used in preventing the common cold and for high-stress conditions.

Deficiency: Scurvy (a disease of deficient collagen that appears as bleeding from all mucosal surfaces, gum bleeding, tooth loss, and skin sores), fatigue, drastic behavioral changes, gum swelling and bleeding.

Overuse: Nausea, vomiting, heartburn, abdominal cramps, and gastrointestinal upset, fatigue, headache, diarrhea. May lead to the formation of urinary tract stones. Individuals with a history of oxalate kidney stones should monitor their vitamin C intake.

Interactions: May increase the absorption of chromium and iron (from plant sources), and interfere with absorption of copper. Its use in chemotherapy is controversial.

Relationship to Chakras: Primary chakra: root. Secondary chakras: throat, third eye, crown. Vitamin C is a classic supplement for the root chakra, because it supports the body's defenses via the adrenal glands, by the production of stress hormones, by its support of the immune system, and by its antioxidant action. Also, it is typically found in foods that are red, such as cranberries and other red berries, making it particularly appropriate for the red vibration of the root chakra. If the root chakra is not in balance, eating more vitamin C-rich foods or taking a vitamin C supplement may help bring our feeling of being protected and grounded back into balance. The throat chakra resonates with vitamin C due to its function in maintaining healthy gums. Vitamin C is linked to the third eye chakra through its role in assisting in making neurotransmitters in the brain, and to the crown chakra because of its importance for nerve cells.

Vitamin D (cholecalciferol, ergocalciferol, the "sunshine" vitamin)
Description and Sources: A fat-soluble vitamin, often touted to be hormonelike in its action. Vitamin D can be made when sunlight interacts with the skin or when we eat fatty fish, eggs from hens given vitamin D in their feed, or fortified foods (such as milk, yogurt, cereals).

Functions: Regulates levels of calcium and phosphorus in the body. Improves bone health and impacts immune system activity.

Intake: To prevent vitamin D deficiency and rickets (which leads to bone softening and deformity), the National Academy of Sciences recommends 200 units (5 micrograms) for individuals from birth through fifty years of age, and 400 units (10 micrograms) for those older than fifty years of age. However, higher daily doses (800 to 1,000 units) have been recommended for older adults for bone health. Keep in mind that the amount of vitamin D you get naturally through your skin may change throughout the year with varying periods of sunlight, and, therefore, alter your dietary supplement requirement. Populations that live in northern latitudes with less sun exposure tend to need more vitamin D from food or supplemental forms.

Deficiency: Rickets, muscle pain, fatigue. Possible increased risk for cancer, autoimmune disease, hypertension, and diabetes.

Overuse: Excess calcium in the body, resulting in weakness, fatigue, headache, nausea, gastrointestinal symptoms, dizziness, pain in muscle and bone.

Interactions: Vitamin D supplementation may increase intestinal absorption of magnesium. Exercise caution when using vitamin D in conjunction with drugs or supplements that increase calcium levels in the body.

Relationship to Chakras: Primary chakra: root. Secondary chakras: throat, third eye, crown. Vitamin D speaks to the coordination of the major body systems by the root and crown chakras. Since this vitamin carries the sunlight vibration, it brings in a high frequency resonant with the crown chakra. This vibration is felt throughout the entire organism at the cellular level; every cell has a receptor for vitamin D. With this balance in place, the neurotransmitters (third eye chakra) shift into a higher frequency, and a better mood results. Vitamin D also feeds the parathyroid glands, which are connected to the throat chakra.

MINERALS

Calcium

Description and Sources: Chalky, white compound found in milk products, green vegetables (kale and broccoli, for example), and canned fish with bones.

Functions: Widespread in the body (the majority—about ninety-nine percent—is in bone, but it is also in blood, extracellular fluid, and muscle).

Used for a variety of functions, including nerve transmission, muscle contraction, blood-vessel activity, and transport of substances in and out of the cell. Needed for bone mineralization. Used to treat rickets and osteoporosis.

Intake: Postmenopausal women who are prone to increases in bone loss may benefit from calcium supplementation: 1,000 to 1,600 milligrams elemental calcium has been used to prevent osteoporosis in this population. Additionally, calcium supplementation would be potentially suitable for lactose-intolerant individuals and vegetarians who do not consume dairy products.

Deficiency: Bone demineralization, premenstrual syndrome (PMS), hypertension, stroke, heart conditions.

Overuse: Hypercalcemia (high blood levels of calcium), kidney stones, arterial calcification, possible increased risk of prostate cancer.

Interactions: Absorption can be enhanced when calcium is taken together with vitamin D. Calcium supplements at high levels can decrease magnesium, iron, zinc uptake, so it is advisable to take them separately. Several pharmaceuticals (antibiotics, diuretics, and thyroid drugs) interact with calcium supplementation and can lead to changes in calcium levels in the body. Therefore, if you are taking medications, discuss these potential interactions with your healthcare professional.

Relationship to Chakras: Primary chakra: root. Secondary chakras: sacral, heart, third eye, crown. The density of calcium connects strongly with the root chakra through the mineral's ability to support the body's skeletal framework and its role as part of muscle fibers. Calcium acts as an anchor for the root chakra. Even though there is solidity to calcium that makes it stable, it has another personality that is resonant with the sacral, heart, third eye, and crown chakras: the ability to encourage movement in the body through its effects on the electrical potential of cells, which in turn effects the contraction of muscle, the squeezing of the blood vessels, and the transport of substances in and out of (nerve) cells.

Copper

Description and Sources: Pinkish metal found in a variety of foods, such as organ meats, grains, seafood, beef, and cocoa.

Functions: Serves as a catalyst in many enzymes (called oxidases) in the body. Helps form bone, red blood cells, and proteins like elastin and collagen.

Intake: Patients on hemodialysis may be at higher risk for copper deficiency—supplementation may be beneficial. Copper supplementation (2.5 milligrams daily) has been used together with calcium, zinc, and manganese for preventing bone loss in postmenopausal women. Individuals who have had gastric bypass surgery may be susceptible to low copper levels. Note that some genetic conditions can lead to toxic copper accumulation in the body—check with your healthcare practitioner before taking copper supplements.

Deficiency: Osteoporosis, anemia, baldness, diarrhea, fatigue.

Overuse: Depression, fever, irritability, nausea, joint and muscle pain, vomiting.

Interactions: Iron, vitamin C, and zinc may decrease copper absorption.

Relationship to Chakras: Primary chakra: root. The root chakra is known for its slow, dense energy. Copper orchestrates this energy movement by playing a role in the intricate interactions among cells, particularly those cells belonging to the root chakra, like bone, blood, and muscle cells, and by helping to build proteins and support tissue.

Iron

Description and Sources: Grayish metal found abundantly in earth's crust and in foods such as meats and vegetables. The highest amounts are in beef, liver, and lamb; moderate amounts are in other animal meats, like pork and poultry, and in beans.

Functions: Assists in the transfer of oxygen and carbon dioxide in the blood through hemoglobin and in the muscle through myoglobin. Plays a significant role in energy production and utilization.

Intake: Supplemental high dose iron (50 to 100 milligrams three times daily) has been used to treat iron-deficiency anemia. Vegetarians and athletes have increased iron needs. Low stomach acid production, which commonly occurs with age, may also lead to lower iron absorption. Iron supplementation can also potentially help with improving cognition and for attention deficit disorder in individuals with iron deficiency.

Deficiency: Anemia, fatigue, cognitive impairment, hair loss.

Overuse: Stomach irritation and pain, diarrhea or constipation, nausea, vomiting.

Interactions: Calcium, soy protein, and zinc may impair iron absorption. Vitamin C improves the absorption of iron from plant sources. Iron supplements may interfere with antibiotics and thyroid medication.

Relationship to Chakras: Primary chakra: root. Iron is one the main elements found in the earth's crust. Due to its dense, earth-energy vibration, iron is one of the most nourishing substances for the root chakra and physical body. In its pure form, it is a lustrous metallic color, but when oxidized, it converts to a reddish color. The combination of iron and oxygen gives blood its deep red color. These two substances together allow humans to have energy to live fully and deeply and thus take in the earth experience. Low iron levels translate to a lifeless body. However, too much iron in the body can be toxic for organs like the heart and the liver, especially for those individuals with a genetic susceptibility called hemochromatosis, which is storing high amounts of iron. Menstruating women who lose iron in their monthly blood flow, and who do not eat iron-rich foods may need to stabilize their root chakra with the anchor of iron.

Phosphorus (phosphates)

Description and Sources: Element present in a variety of foods, including grains, vegetables, dairy products, animal products, and legumes.

Functions: Phosphorus is a core component of much of the body, comprising (1) part of the phospholipids that compose the cell membrane, (2) the genetic DNA and RNA material, and (3) the energy currency (adenosine triphosphate, or ATP) used in the body. It is needed for bone and tooth formation, for heart muscle and kidney function, and for vitamins to be able to convert food to energy.

Intake: Phosphorus supplements are not common because of the ubiquity of phosphorus in the diet. However, they can be used for individuals with low phosphate levels in the blood or for those with calcium-containing kidney stones.

Deficiency: Muscle and nerve dysfunction, anxiety, bone pain, fatigue, irregular breathing, numbness, skin sensitivity, weakness.

Overuse: Potential negative impact on bone mineral density.

Interactions: Bile sequestrants and antacids that contain aluminum, calcium and/or magnesium can bind phosphate and prevent its absorption in the gut, eventually resulting in low blood phosphate. High phosphorus can decrease gut absorption of iron, copper, and zinc. Some anticonvulsants lower blood phosphate levels. Individuals with kidney disease should avoid high amounts of phosphorus. Additionally, medications that effect electrolytes (for example, diuretics, potassium-containing agents) may alter body levels of phosphate. Excessive calcium may interfere with phosphate activity.

Relationship to Chakras: Primary chakra: root. Secondary chakras: sacral, solar plexus, third eye. Phosphorus is embedded throughout every cell of the body connecting it with the basic energy of the root chakra. Since it is associated with the lipid cell membranes in the form of phospholipids (fats attached to phosphorus), it resonates closely with the sacral chakra's function of moving materials in and out of cells. It also resonates with the third eye chakra, since many fats in the brain are phospholipids. The fact that phosphorus is part of ATP, which is found ubiquitously in the body, indicates that it is essential for the exchange of energy, a function overseen by the solar plexus chakra.

Selenium

See chapter on the sacral chakra for more details. Selenium supplementation has been shown to be helpful in reducing cancer (except skin) risk (see the chapter on the sacral chakra)—most notably prostate cancer incidence. Individuals who most benefit from supplementation are those with lower prostate specific antigen (PSA, a protein made by the prostate gland, can be measured in the blood; high amounts may be indicative of cancer) and lower selenium levels. The typical dose is 200 micrograms daily.

Zinc

Description and Sources: A bluish gray metal found abundantly in the earth's crust and in foods such as oysters, animal products, beans, nuts, grains, and seeds.

Functions: Required for the synthesis of protein, DNA and RNA, prostate-gland function, immune system regulation, wound healing, cell growth, taste and smell, skin health, bone formation, and for the activity of more than 300 enzymes (proteins) in the body.

Intake: Individuals with gastrointestinal disorders that result in nutrient malabsorption (like ulcerative colitis, Crohn's disease, or even diarrhea) can have low zinc due to reduced absorption. Vegetarians may benefit from zinc supplementation since animal foods contain more bioavailable zinc than plant foods (plant foods contain compounds called phytates which prevent zinc from being absorbed in the gut). Those who want to facilitate wound healing, such as in chronic leg ulcers, may be helped by zinc supplementation. The studies on taking zinc for the common cold reveal mixed results.

Deficiency: Growth retardation, mental lethargy, low sperm count, hair loss, skin dryness and acne, slow wound healing, impaired thyroid function and insulin action, decreased sense of smell and taste.

Overuse: Nausea, vomiting, metallic taste in mouth, copper deficiency, gastrointestinal symptoms (such as diarrhea and stomach upset), and fatigue.

Interactions: Calcium can inhibit zinc absorption in the gut—take these two supplements separately. High supplemental levels of zinc may decrease copper absorption. It has been advised to refrain from taking iron and zinc together on an empty stomach as they may compete for absorption—instead, take them with food to prevent competition. Magnesium and zinc may compete for absorption—take them at different times. Vitamin B2 (riboflavin) may facilitate the absorption of zinc. High-fiber foods may bind zinc and prevent its absorption. Zinc supplementation may interfere with the absorption and activity of antibiotics. Consult your healthcare professional for specifics.

Relationship to Chakras: Primary chakra: root. Secondary chakra: throat. Zinc is vital to the workings of the organs within the root chakra and through its close tie to the functions of protein in the body. Its unique role in taste and smell make it essential to the throat chakra, the residence of many sensory organs.

BOTANICALS/OTHER

Adrenal Support

The root chakra controls the fear response. In the body, this response, ideally suited to assist with short-term emergencies, is wired to the functioning of the adrenal glands. Overstimulation of the adrenal glands and excessive stress hormones utilize significant root chakra energy and causes depleting effects, such as inability to think and learn, disturbed sleep patterns, alterations in appetite, and changes in metabolism. Supporting the adrenals with nutritional products is advised for those individuals who show signs of adrenal fatigue. When we feel completely stressed and tired, on the verge of exhaustion, the chakra circuit will be inclined to assist the root chakra in getting energy in any way possible. For example, our solar plexus chakra may lead us to get quick energy by eating high-sugar snacks to keep going. By doing this, we begin to drain energy from our solar plexus (which becomes imbalanced with sugary snacks) and the organs held within this energetic realm. Long term, we may develop unhealthy blood-sugar fluctuations which could progress to type 2 diabetes. Therefore, depletion of energy from one organ system (and chakra) inevitably leads to a ripple effect where other organs (and chakras) are affected if the initial imbalance is not corrected.

In the instance of adrenal fatigue, choosing botanical products that act as **adaptogens** (herbs that balance the stress responses, thus toning down an overactive adrenal response or fortifying a weakened one) is an option for healing the hormone-immune response or harmonizing solar plexus and root chakra energies. Some of these botanical products include dang shen *(Codonopsis pilosula),* eleuthero root *(Eleutherococcus senticosus),* licorice *(Glycyrrhiza glabra*), holy basil *(Ocinum sanctum),* ginseng *(Panax ginseng),* rhodiola *(Rhodiola rosea),* schisandra *(Schisandra chinensis),* ashwagandha *(Withania somnifera),* cordyceps *(Cordyceps sinensis),* and reishi mushroom *(Ganoderma lucidum).* Using supplements with adaptogenic properties in conjunction with lifestyle techniques, such as stress reduction, can help to dig the root chakra out of a ditch filled with fear, stress, and worry. As part of this strategy, it may be valuable to engage the root chakra in a dialogue on what the body feels that it needs to constantly be running from or battling against. Understanding the reason(s) for the constant fight-or-flight response may present solutions for reducing the baseline of alarm.

Anti-Inflammation

With excessive root chakra energy, the body may become inflamed, embodying the classical signs of redness, pain, and heat. Classical inflammatory symptoms involving root-chakra physiology include the joints becoming painful and swollen, or the skin becoming irritated. In fact, many chronic conditions today, like obesity, type 2 diabetes, and heart disease, are thought to have an underlying inflammation component. Pharmaceuticals that cool the body of the inflammatory processes also have serious side effects, such as gastric bleeding and stomach upset within a short time after taking them. So natural products become even more desirable, although they may also have some precautions regarding their use.

Questions to ask your root chakra under conditions of inflammation are: What about life makes me so 'heated'? Why is my energy erupting into a volcaniclike response? How can I best be calmed and cooled?

Cat's claw *(Uncaria tomentosa):* The inner bark and roots of this plant have been used for their anti-inflammatory, antioxidant, and immune-stimulating effects. After one week of use, cat's claw relieved knee pain related to physical activity. It may improve symptoms related to rheumatoid arthritis. Taking specific preparations of this plant in extract form, at 100 milligrams to 180 milligrams (60 milligrams in three divided doses) daily, has been shown to be effective for reducing pain in individuals with knee osteoarthritis and rheumatoid arthritis, respectively. Side effects include headaches, dizziness, and vomiting. Cat's claw may lead to a worsening of motor symptoms in neurological disorders (such as Parkinson's disease). Avoid using it with immunosuppressants or blood pressure-lowering supplements or drugs. It should not be taken during pregnancy.

Hops *(Humulus lupulus):*Certain hop extracts have been shown to cool down the inflammatory cascade in the body, resulting in pain relief from conditions such as osteoarthritis.

Indian frankincense *(Boswellia serrata):* This gum resin, used in traditional Ayurvedic medicine, has been used as an anti-inflammatory and antiarthritic, and has been used for asthma. For arthritic conditions, 1,000 milligrams (taken as 333 milligrams three times daily) and 3,600 milligrams daily have been used for osteo- and rheumatoid arthritis, respectively. A study published in 2008 indicated that 250 milligrams of a novel boswellia extract, enriched with a specific boswellic acid, resulted in decreased pain and improved function after just one week of use by osteoarthritic individuals. Boswellia has also been used for inflammatory gut conditions and asthma. Gastrointestinal effects such as pain, heartburn, nausea, and diarrhea may be experienced while taking this supplement.

Willow bark *(Salix alba)*: The willow tree, native to parts of Europe and Asia, has been used since the time of Hippocrates (fifth century B.C.) for its bark, which produces anti-inflammatory effects. The active compound, salicin, converts in the body into salicylic acid, the same compound found in aspirin. These compounds have pain-relieving, anti-inflammatory, antifever actions similar to those of aspirin; however, ingesting salicin and salicylic acid, just like ingesting aspirin, may also lead to gastrointestinal side effects. Due to its ability to influence blood clotting, this botanical should not be taken in conjunction with anticoagulant supplements or drugs. Short-term use of this plant is advocated. A willow-bark extract containing 120 to 240 milligrams of salicin has been taken to reduce back pain, and a greater degree of relief was experienced at the higher (240 milligrams) dose. Do not take if you are allergic to salicylates. Side effects include itching and rash.

Joint Support

Stuck, stagnant energy in the matrix of the root chakra can lead to brittle, depleted, and inflamed bones. If you experience joint issues, ask yourself what is preventing you from moving forward or what is keeping you stuck in the past. Utilizing the support of various nutrients can help rebuild the joint cartilage and thus prevent further degradation.

Glucosamine sulfate: Glucosamine, made from the simple carbohydrate glucose and the amino acid glutamine, is found naturally throughout the body, but especially within the joints. In supplemental form as glucosamine sulfate, it may help with symptoms of osteoarthritis, including providing pain relief and better functioning, by rebuilding joint cartilage. Side effects include gastrointestinal discomfort and increased blood sugar. The supplement form is derived from the exoskeletons of shellfish or produced synthetically. Do not take together with anticoagulant supplements or drugs, as its effects may be enhanced and it may cause bleeding or bruising. For osteoarthritis, 1,500 milligrams can be taken daily or taken in three divided doses (sometimes in combination with chondroitin sulfate, 400 milligrams three times daily); for knee pain due to previous injury, 2,000 milligrams glucosamine hydrochloride has been shown to be effective in reducing pain and improving function.

Chondroitin sulfate: Like glucosamine, chondroitin sulfate exists in the body as a part of cartilage structure. These long carbohydrate chains keep cartilage flexible and prevent degeneration by blocking the activity of specific enzymes known to degrade cartilage. Supplemental chondroitin sulfate (typically made from shark cartilage or cow trachea cartilage) at a dose of 200 to 400 milligrams two to three times daily, or 1000 to 1200 milligrams in a single dose, may be helpful in treating osteoarthritis. Often, joint health supplements will include both glucosamine sulfate and chondroitin sulfate. Overall, chondroitin sulfate is well-tolerated, although a variety of side effects have been reported in clinical trials where chondroitin was used: stomach pain, eyelid swelling, hair loss, nausea, and changes in bowel pattern, to name a few. These effects may or may not be associated with chondroitin supplementation. Do not take together with anticoagulants. Do not take if you have asthma, as it may exacerbate symptoms. Men with prostate cancer or an increased risk of prostate cancer should avoid this supplement.

Methylsulfonylmethane (MSM): This sulfur-containing compound, found in plants and animals, is used for a wide array of body functions, but primarily for joint health. Animal studies suggest it might help to decrease joint degradation. Side effects include nausea, gastrointestinal discomfort, headache, fatigue, insomnia, itching, and allergic-type reactions. The common dose range is 500 milligrams three times daily, up to 3 grams twice daily. It is often used in conjunction with glucosamine sulfate. Its use in allergic rhinitis is also being explored (see chapter on the throat chakra).

Immune Support
The plants or botanically-based actives listed below have been used to bring the immune system into a state of balance—in many cases, through

stimulation of immunity. The immune system can be thrown into imbalance by a variety of factors, including undue stress, little sleep, poor diet, and inactivity. When we deplete our internal reserves without having sufficient root-chakra energy, our defenses run low, and we are susceptible to attack by external invaders. These plants help the root chakra to reclaim its energy by heightening the response of the innate immune system. They could be seen as boosters for the root chakra. Immune system issues may signal that you need to work on your sense of boundaries and how you discern what is self and what is not self. They may also indicate that you need to give greater support to what you stand for in the physical world or a firm yes or no answer in a situation that is presenting itself.

For those individuals with a hypervigilant immune system, such as those with autoimmune disease, supplementation with these plants may be contraindicated. Concomitant use with immunosuppressant drugs is also not recommended. Since these botanicals are so potent in their immune effects, it may be worthwhile to take them for short periods of time (about four to six weeks), with some time before the next cycle of supplementation. Finally, several of these medicinal plants and plant parts need to be taken at the start of a cold or flu.

Andrographis *(Andrographis paniculata):* Plant commonly grown in India and other parts of Asia. The leaves and roots have been used for their antibiotic, antiallergy, and immune-stimulating properties. Commonly taken for colds, infections, HIV/AIDS, allergies, and depressed immune function. Side effects include itching, fatigue, headache, diarrhea, nausea, vomiting, heartburn, gastrointestinal discomfort, and anaphylactic reactions. Pregnant women should not use andrographis due to its potential abortifacient effects. Do not take with supplements or drugs that have anticoagulant, blood pressure-lowering, or immunosuppressive actions. Individuals with autoimmune disease should not take this supplement, due to its potential immune-stimulating effects. Various andrographis extracts have been used for preventing the onset or shortening the duration of the common cold. Take at the onset of a cold and continue for several days. Andrographis is best used for short durations (four to five days).

Astragalus *(Astragalus membranaceus):* Flowering plant typically used for the common cold and upper respiratory infections, wound healing, injuries, immune system strengthening, viral infections, chronic fatigue syndrome, and fibromyalgia. Cell studies indicate that it can improve the immune response by stimulating the activity of immune cells. Even though a wide range of doses has been used (1 to 30 grams daily), the typical dose for enhancing immune function is 4 to 7 grams. Doses larger than 28 grams daily may cause suppression of the immune system.

Echinacea *(Echinachea purpurea):* Also called purple coneflower, echinacea has long been used by Native Americans for medicinal purposes. Nowadays, echinacea supplementation is advised to prevent the common cold and to assist in the recovery from upper respiratory infections. Although it may reduce the symptoms of the common cold by 10 to 30 percent in some studies, other studies show that taking echinacea products has no effect. Side effects are varied and include nausea, vomiting, allergic reactions (such as rash, tingling, and/or numb tongue), bowel-pattern changes, headache, and dizziness. It may interact with the metabolism of several drugs (including caffeine); if you are taking any drugs, consult with a practitioner before taking echinacea. A wide variety of doses has been taken, depending on the preparation (capsules, juice, tea, tincture).

Elderberry *(Sambucus nigra):* The elderberry fruit is concentrated with numerous plant compounds that function as antiviral, antioxidant, and immune-stimulating agents. Elderberry has been shown to reduce the duration of influenza symptoms by more than fifty percent. A common formulation is elderberry-juice syrup. Side effects include weakness, dizziness, numbness, stupor, and allergic reactions (particularly in people with a grass-pollen allergy).

Prostate Health

The prostate gland, found in men only, provides storage for seminal fluid; as a result, the root chakra is seen as the creative center for men (for women, the creative center is the sacral chakra). A man's creativity is often seen as connected with the elements of survival (such as his career). When creativity becomes blocked or when root chakra energy becomes stagnant due to issues concerning family, job, or money, prostatic conditions such as prostate-gland enlargement (benign prostatic hyperplasia, or BPH) or inflammation (prostatitis) may occur. Prostate issues may require men to more closely examine how they express creativity in their lives. Having an occupation that allows one's creative nature to unfold may be one means to a healthy prostate.

Lycopene: Lycopene is a red-colored carotenoid found in fruits and vegetables, such as pink grapefruit, watermelon, and tomato. Unlike other carotenoids (such as beta-carotene), it does not convert to vitamin A once ingested. In addition to its ability to protect cells as an antioxidant, cell studies indicate that it inhibits cancer-cell proliferation. In general, low lycopene in the blood and/or tissues appears to be related to incidence of prostate cancer, although there is a cell study that shows that lycopene worsens metastasis (spread of cancer) in a prostate-cell line. Supplementation studies have resulted in positive benefits in men with prostate cancer: 4 milligrams of lycopene twice daily delayed or prevented progression to prostate cancer in men with a precursor of prostate cancer, and 15 milligrams twice daily for three weeks decreased prostate-tumor growth in men with prostate cancer. Although there are some exceptions, in general, populations that eat greater amounts of tomato products (which contain lycopene) or that have higher amounts of lycopene in the blood have decreased risk of prostate cancer compared with those that eat less dietary sources of lycopene and have less lycopene in their blood.

Due to its red color, its association with the prostate gland, and its antioxidant potential, lycopene resonates strongly with the root chakra. However, because it protects lipid membranes and has been considered an anticancer agent, it also connects to the sacral chakra. The heart chakra is also implicated because of lycopene's significant impact on the organs in this energetic area, including the heart and lungs (see chapter on the heart chakra). Studies show that those who supplement their diets with lycopene, and populations that eat more dietary sources of lycopene, have reduced cardiovascular risk. Supplementation with lycopene may also help reduce the symptoms of exercise-induced asthma. Because of the strong influence on the root and heart chakras, lycopene is an important energetic substance for men, linking their root chakra survival needs to their heart's passion.

Phytosterols: *See the heart chakra chapter for specific details.* Natural plant compounds called phytosterols can be included into foods or supplemented daily to benefit prostate health. Amounts of 60 to 130 milligrams, divided into two to three doses daily, have been studied for this purpose.

Saw palmetto *(Serenoa repens):* Whole berry or berry extracts of saw palmetto have been used to treat BPH because of saw palmetto's actions on testosterone metabolism and its ability to slow proliferative prostate growth. Saw palmetto is generally well tolerated, but may cause gastrointestinal effects, dizziness, and headaches in some individuals. It is not to be taken in conjunction with anticoagulant supplements or drugs. For BPH, supplementation with a lipophilic (fat-containing) saw palmetto extract containing eighty to ninety percent fatty acids has been used at 160 milligrams twice daily or 320 milligrams once daily.

CHAPTER 5

SUPPLEMENTS FOR CREATIVITY AND FLOW (SACRAL CHAKRA)

There can be no transforming of darkness into light and of apathy into movement without emotion.
CARL GUSTAV JUNG

CHAKRA DESCRIPTION

To balance the solid nature of the root chakra, we have an opposite vibration in close proximity—one that is in motion, always changing with the flux of creativity and emotion we may feel in our exchanges with others. Whereas the root chakra gets us to dig our heels into the mud of living, the sacral chakra gives us permission to dance and play, enjoying the pleasures of life in a childlike way, especially through expression of our creative self and through the evolution and unfolding of partnership. The sacral chakra transitions our energy from one of tribe into one encompassing *duality*—masculine/feminine, yin/yang, sun/moon—within ourselves and allows us to honor one another in the commitment of relationship. It honors the movement of the body in flowing forms, throughout the body. Any part of us associated with or responding to water or fats hooks us to this part of ourselves.

Words associated with the sacral chakra: *Balance, chaos, creativity, duality, emotions, experience, flow, fluidity, movement, orange, partnership, pleasure, relationships, sexuality, water.*

CHAKRA ANATOMY AND PHYSIOLOGY

The sacral chakra endows us with a fluid, ever-changing, creative, dynamic capacity and, its energy, in the form of water, pervades our bodies and planet. This vibration is responsible for ensuring the flow of materials in and out of the cell, and for the fluid that bathes them and within which they survive (called the extracellular matrix). The fence of slippery fats surrounding the cell (known as the cell membrane) is the guarded territory of the sacral chakra. Water and liquid fats possess the ability to ease the passage of substances through the rigid structure formed by the root chakra. The strength of flowing substances comes from their ability to adapt and yield. The undulation of creativity and of the life experience, felt through the senses, weaves in and out of the continuum of our fluid being.

Sacral chakra anatomy: Bladder, extra- and intercellular water, hips, kidneys, large intestine/colon, ovaries, uterus.

HEALTHY INDICATIONS

A person who is comfortable with their emotional, sensing self is someone who manifests their creative potential, expresses emotions, goes with the flow of life, lives their life's dream, maintains healthy relationships with others, honors their uniqueness, and has fun by engaging in pleasurable activities.

UNHEALTHY INDICATIONS

If you answer yes to a majority of these questions, your sacral chakra may need healing:

- *Do you feel stuck or unable to express emotions and creativity?* The sign of a sacral chakra imbalance is the feeling of stagnation, an inability to move to action in one's life. Often, individuals with sacral chakra imbalance have difficulty in recovering from deep, emotionally traumatic issues, and as a result, their lives feel barren. These individuals are prone to emotional eating since they do not feel their feelings—they stuff them down with foods and constant eating instead. Their physiology tends to be either too swollen or too dehydrated, indicating impaired control of fluids in the body.

- *Do you feel unsatisfied in your relationships with others?* Have you been in relationships that are not equal and contain a degree of uncertainty or instability? Do you allow yourself to be emotionally abused? Is commitment to a relationship or a creative project an ongoing struggle? Follow-through is a growth area for individuals with sacral chakra issues. Typically, they are strong at coming up with ideas or starting a relationship, living in the high of the initial creative burst or romantic flair, but then their initiations fall flat: the idea remains unimplemented and the relationship fizzles out. They eventually succumb to the idea that "I am not a creative person" or "I'd rather be alone," denying their ability to come full circle with any aspect of life other than the repetition of this debilitating pattern.

- *Do you have issues revolving around sexuality?* Or, for women, medical issues with reproductive organs (for example, the uterus or ovaries)? The sacral chakra harbors our life pattern and beliefs around sex and what it means to be creative. Imbalance may manifest as meaningless sexual encounters, abstinence, or fear around sexuality, and could stem from traumatic experiences or dysfunctional family patterns that have been passed on through the energetic lineage.

SUPPLEMENTS FOR THE SACRAL CHAKRA

MACRONUTRIENTS AND MACRONUTRIENT SUPPLEMENTS

Fat

Just as protein provides a building block-like structure for the root chakra, fat sculpts a soft framework that the body can use to flow through experiences and emotions. Unfortunately, fat has been a maligned nutrient for many years. Paralleling the denial of fat in the American diet is the inability to experience joy and pleasure. Think back to the advent of low-fat foods in the early 1990s and how at the same time, throughout that entire decade, we became an increasingly overworked, overburdened society with no time to reap the pleasure of the abundance that comes from working. Because we've succumbed to the fat taboo within the past two decades, it is no wonder that there has been an increase in obesity; from an energy perspective, the starvation of the sacral chakra may have led to strain in the solar plexus chakra because we are eating carbohydrates in place of fats.

In the end, without the flexibility imparted by fat, we become rigid and depleted at the same time. The body attempts to establish flow by creating its own fat, albeit in dysfunctional and excessive ways ("belly fat"). Two decades later, we find ourselves in an obesity crisis.

Rather than low-fat or no-fat approaches to eating, the sacral chakra craves a balance of healthy fats. The nutritional spotlight needs to swing from the *quantity* of fat to the *quality* of fat. The quality of fat in the current supply of high-sugar, high-fat, processed foods is low; these fats are synthetically derived through the process known as hydrogenation. The resulting trans fats enable a product to live a longer shelf life, but our bodies to live a shorter life. When we eat these synthetic fats, the body (and higher chakras like the heart chakra) rejects these fats by exhibiting high "bad" cholesterol and low "good" cholesterol.

In addition to the copious quantities of trans fat in their diet, Americans are also eating too many omega-6 fats from vegetable oils, like corn oil. Offsetting the balance of fats in the body, especially the omega-6 to omega-3 fat ratio, can put us into a state of inflammation, or "body on fire." Corn revs the fiery nature of the solar plexus, and excessively eating products made from corn (such as corn oil, corn syrup solids, and high-fructose corn syrup) taxes the solar plexus chakra. Without the cooling fats from the sea, the omega-3 fats, we can find ourselves with any number of inflammatory conditions. One way to balance the warming (solar plexus fire) and cooling (sacral water) ratio of fats in the body is to eat more omega-3 fats from fish, leafy greens, nuts, and seeds. Since these foods are not part of many people's diets in appreciable amounts, omega-3 supplements are available.

Fish oils: If there is one supplement that harmonizes with the sacral chakra most completely, it would be fish oil, which is comprised primarily of the fatty acids known as eicosapentaenoic acid (EPA) and docosahexaenoic acid (DHA). Not only do fish live in the soothing water element that is resonant with the sacral chakra, but they also contain oils that are ideal for the flowing movement of the human body. The purity of a fish oil supplement is important to consider, since the supply of fish can be tainted with the high level of methylmercury found in ocean waters. For best results, check to be sure your fish oil supplement does not have a fishy taste or smell. These long-chain omega-3 oils are "body-ready," which means that they do not have to undergo further conversion in the body and, as a result, can easily be assimilated throughout several tissues, particularly in the brain and eyes.

Low amounts of these long-chain omega-3 fish oils in the diet have been shown to be associated with a variety of conditions, such as heart disease, inflammation, and behavioral disorders. The American Heart Association recommends about 1 gram of EPA/DHA per day for individuals with heart disease, and a higher dose (2 to 4 grams) for those with high triglycerides. Please note that high doses may lead to excessive bleeding and changes in blood clotting. In the full energy picture, these fats interlace the sacral chakra (also known as the second chakra) to the circuit of its even-numbered counterparts (as well as on through to the crown chakra); through their effects on heart disease, these fats connect the sacral chakra to the heart (fourth) chakra, and through their effects on the brain and behavior and nerves, they connect to the third eye (sixth) and crown (seventh) chakra.

Plant oils (borage-seed oil, evening primrose oil, flaxseed oil): Another source of healthy omega-3 fats comes from flaxseed. Flaxseed oil contains high amounts of the omega-3 fat called alpha-linolenic acid (ALA). ALA is the precursor fat to EPA and DHA. If your body needs EPA and DHA, it has to convert ALA through an extensive metabolic process. This process is not very efficient in most people, since it can be impacted by stress or mineral deficiencies. Indeed, it has been shown that the effects of ALA ingestion are not entirely similar to effects of EPA and DHA ingestion. However, ALA appears to be important for maintaining cardiovascular health. Flaxseed oil supplementation would be an acceptable alternative for those who do not eat fish. Choose organic, cold-pressed sources whenever they are available, and do not subject the oil to heat. Like fish oil, high doses of flaxseed oil could lead to changes in bleeding time.

Two other oils, borage-seed oil and evening primrose oil, are sometimes used for supplementation, although there is debate regarding their
efficacy. Borage-seed oil contains a relatively high level of gamma-linolenic
acid (GLA), an omega-6 fat that is anti-inflammatory. Consequently, supplementation with this oil could have anti-inflammatory effects on joints and
skin conditions. Along similar lines, evening primrose oil contains GLA, although at a lower percentage than borage-seed oil. Like borage-seed oil,
evening primrose oil is thought to help with inflammatory conditions such
as rheumatoid arthritis, eczema, breast pain, and even PMS.

VITAMINS

Vitamin B6 (pyridoxine)

See the solar plexus chakra chapter for full details. Vitamin B6 has been shown to
be useful in reducing PMS symptoms such as breast pain, depression, and
anxiety. There does not appear to be any benefit by taking high doses; therefore, lower doses (50 to 100 milligrams) should be used to reduce risk of
side effects. Vitamin B6 supplementation at 100 milligrams daily was shown
to be as effective as using the drug bromocriptine, without the same degree
of side effects. In combination with magnesium (200 milligrams magnesium
oxide), vitamin B6 (50 milligrams daily) reduced PMS-associated anxiety.

Vitamin E

Description and Sources: Although most supplemental vitamin E is
alpha-tocopherol (d-alpha-tocopherol is the naturally occurring form), vitamin E actually refers to eight different forms of this fat-soluble vitamin, including alpha-, beta-, gamma-, and delta-tocopherols and four tocotrienols.
These yellow oils can be found in unrefined vegetable oils, especially wheat
germ oil, and in seeds, nuts, and grains.

Functions: Just as vitamin C is a protective water-soluble antioxidant,
vitamin E is a lipid-soluble antioxidant that protects fats in the body from
degradation. It also helps maintain the stability and integrity of cell membranes (similar to the role of fats). Each of the individual forms of vitamin E
may have a slightly different function, and more research is being conducted
on their health benefits.

Intake: Those who experience chronic malabsorption of fat such as in cystic fibrosis and Crohn's disease may require a vitamin E supplement. Due to its anticoagulant effects and potential increased risk of bleeding, use with caution before, during, and after surgical procedures (consult your health-care professional).

Deficiency: Tends to be rare, but can occur in those who do not absorb fat or in individuals on a fat-restricted diet. Symptoms include decreased integrity of cell membranes, particularly those of the red blood cells; hemolytic anemia; muscle weakness; neuropathy; infertility; PMS; and increased risk for chronic diseases like cancer, atherosclerosis, and rheumatoid arthritis, to name a few.

Overuse: Fatigue, headache, hemorrhage, blurred vision, rash, gastrointestinal distress, muscle weakness.

Interactions: Do not use in conjunction with supplements or drugs that have anticoagulant activity. If you are using drugs that result in fat malabsorption, such as orlistat or cholestyramine, you may experience reduced uptake of vitamin E by the gut. High doses of vitamin E may affect the physiological actions of vitamins A and K. Furthermore, vitamin E supplements may increase the metabolism of specific drugs, amplifying their effects.

Relationship to Chakras: Primary chakra: sacral. Secondary chakras: heart, third eye, crown. Vitamin E is the energetic protector of the fats in the body. When we are unable to support our inherent need to flow, an unstable structure can result, particularly in the areas fed by the lower sacral chakra and by the heart, third eye, and crown chakras.

MINERALS

Calcium

See the root chakra chapter for details. Like magnesium, calcium is present in a variety of tissues, including the extracellular fluid. Women who eat more calcium-rich foods tend to have reduced PMS symptoms. Calcium supplementation of 1,200 to 1,600 milligrams daily (depending on dietary intake) has been recommended as a treatment option for women with PMS. A study in which women with PMS took 1,000 milligrams of calcium for three months revealed that these women experienced less water retention and pain, and fewer mood disturbances than when they took a placebo.

Magnesium

See the heart chakra chapter for details. Magnesium is found within the fluid that bathes cells and, as a result, is connected to the transport of substances from cell to cell. Through its role in helping the body to flow, it is associated with the essence of the sacral chakra. It is also related to the sacral chakra through its ability to improve PMS. Daily magnesium doses of 200 to 360 milligrams have been shown to reduce PMS symptoms such as fluid retention and mood changes (see the third eye chakra chapter).

Selenium

Description and Sources: Metallic substance in foods such as nuts (especially Brazil nuts), crab, liver, fish, poultry, and wheat.

Functions: Prevents the breakdown of fats, especially when combined with vitamin E. Helps to prevent the formation of certain tumors (such as prostate tumors; see the root chakra chapter). Needed for the functioning of specific proteins in body and for the production of thyroid hormones (see throat chakra chapter).

Intake: Individuals with higher body levels of selenium have been shown to be at reduced risk of cancer. Supplementation with 200 micrograms selenium daily decreased cancer incidence by 25 percent.

Deficiency: Cancer, high cholesterol, heart disease, exhaustion, growth impairment, infections.

Overuse: Garlic-smelling breath, nausea, vomiting, abdominal pain, fatigue, irritability, hair loss, skin eruptions and/or yellowing, muscle tenderness, tremor.

Interactions: Vitamin C and zinc may reduce selenium absorption. Do not use together with supplements or drugs that have anticoagulant effects.

Relationship to Chakras: Primary chakra: sacral. Secondary chakras: root, throat. Selenium nourishes the sacral chakra in two ways: by working as a partner with vitamin E to protect the integrity of fats and by harmonizing the chakra's energy flow through selenium's anticancer effects.

Selenium's positive impact on the immune system and on prostate health particularily resonates with the root chakra. Selenium bridges the gap between these lower chakras and the throat chakra through its role in thyroid-gland function.

BOTANICALS/OTHER

Urinary Support

The sacral chakra oversees body tissues concerned with the water element. The primary organs concerned with water balance in the body are the kidneys and urinary tract, which assist the body with removing excess fluid and toxins. The proper functioning of these organs impacts the whole of the system, including the body's electrolyte level, muscle contractions, nerve transmission, blood pressure, and the pH of body compartments (for example, like the blood, saliva, gut). Some issues for these organs can arise from the accumulation of microorganisms within the urinary tract. However, specific nutrients can prevent this buildup and keep bacteria from adhering to the tract.

When you are presented with urinary-tract conditions, it may be useful to reflect on the following questions: What toxins—emotional, mental, or physical—need to flow through me? What emotional excesses am I not willing to let go of? How can I tap into the reservoir of creativity within me? Am I confronted with fear?

Cranberry extract: Extracts of the cranberry fruit and cranberry juice are notorious for their ability to prevent bacteria from adhering to the urinary tract. As a result, they may be helpful for urinary tract infections. The cranberry fruit contains a number of plant compounds to acidify the urine. In people with spinal cord injury and bladder dysfunction, supplementation with cranberry extract tablets for one year significantly reduced the incidence of urinary tract infections. Note that cranberry juice and extract may interfere with the metabolism of a number of drugs. Do not take them in conjunction with supplements or herbs that have anticoagulant activity (especially warfarin). Avoid juices that contain added sugars.

Bearberry _(Uva ursi)_: Uva ursi leaf contains a number of actives, including the bitter agent arbutin, which support its activity as a urinary antiseptic and potentially as a diuretic, making bearberry beneficial for some kidney and bladder conditions. It may protect the uterus and strengthen heart muscle. It is not recommended for pregnant or lactating women, or for children. This botanical should be taken in the short term and under the supervision of a qualified healthcare professional. It can turn urine greenish brown and cause gastric distress and even liver toxicity in some individuals.

Hormonal Support

The sacral chakra is the hub for much hormone activity, particularly in women. Hormone imbalances may give rise to several conditions that can involve other chakras: PMS (third eye chakra), breast pain (heart chakra), and menopausal symptoms (heart and third eye chakras). Typically, plant estrogens (called *phytoestrogens*) have been used as weak estrogens in the body. By blocking the strong effects of the body's estrogen, plant estrogens blunt the physiological effects that result when estrogen binds to cell receptors. Or they enhance a weak estrogenic effect that comes from the absence of estrogen (such as in menopause). Since they work like estrogens, they may have effects on other parts of the body, such as bone or neurotransmitters. Because of phytoestrogens' estrogenlike actions, individuals with a history of hormone-sensitive cancers (which indicate excessive sacral chakra energy) are advised not to take supplements containing phytoestrogens.

Hormonal imbalances require that we examine our internal balance of the feminine and masculine elements. Regardless of whether we are a man or woman, we embody both feminine elements, such as receptivity, warmth, sensitivity, intuition, and grace, and masculine features, like assertiveness, independence, authority, analysis, and leadership. If you have hormonal issues that require healing, reflect on the dynamics between your feminine and masculine natures. Are they balanced or too overly exaggerated in one direction? Are you able to access either of these natures, or does one aspect feel more stifled than the other? Examining these aspects may illuminate the root of your physiological disorders involving the hormones.

Black cohosh *(Cimicifuga racemosa)*: The root of this North American native plant has been found to reduce menopausal symptoms, particularly hot flashes. It has also been used traditionally for inducing labor, and preliminary studies suggest it may also favorably impact bone health. Side effects include gastrointestinal upset, rash, headache, weight gain, breast tenderness, and vaginal bleeding. In some cases, liver damage has been reported. Since it may affect the metabolism of a variety of drugs, consult your healthcare provider before using it, if you are taking any medications. Women with a history of breast cancer or with breast cancer should avoid using. Whether it could affect hormone-sensitive cancers is unknown. Supplementing with a black cohosh extract of 40 milligrams daily has been used in a number of studies to treat menopausal complaints.

Chasteberry fruit *(Vitex agnus-castus):* This fruit has been used for an array of hormone-related menstrual complaints, including PMS, breast pain, and painful menses. Individuals taking it should be aware that its influence on hormones and neurotransmitters may result in interactions with drugs that influence these substances. Also, it has been advised that those with hormone-sensitive conditions (such as a history of breast, ovarian, or endometrial cancers) avoid taking this botanical. Side effects include gastrointestinal complaints, headache, itching, rash, acne, insomnia, and irregular menstrual bleeding. A wide range of doses has been used, and the dose will depend on the unique formulation.

Indole-3-carbinol (I3C)/diindolylmethane (DIM): Indole-3-carbinol (I3C) is a constituent of cruciferous vegetables (like broccoli and brussels sprouts). When I3C is ingested and exposed to stomach acid, it converts into a number of active metabolites, including DIM (diindolylmethane). Supplementation with I3C (and DIM) has been used to balance hormones and to prevent various types of cancers, including breast, cervical, and endometrial cancer). I3C has been shown to be effective in the regression of cervical dysplasia (abnormal cells in the cervix) in a significant percentage of individuals with this abnormality. More clinical research exists for I3C than for DIM. There is controversial discussion about whether it can promote tumor formation in those who are in the initial stage of cancer development. Side effects include skin rash and, in rare instances, elevations in liver enzymes. The common dose for cervical dysplasia and hormone balance is 200 to 400 milligrams daily, and the lower dose works as well as the higher dose in some cases.

Red clover *(Trifolium pratense);* The flowers of red clover have been used for a variety of gynecological complaints, including menopausal symptoms, hot flashes, breast pain, and PMS. Red clover contains isoflavones, which have weak estrogenic effects and modulate estrogen activity. Side effects include rash, headache, and nausea. Do not take it with supplements or drugs that have anticoagulant activity. Since it may alter the metabolism of several drugs, consult with your healthcare provider before using it, if you are on medication. Specifically, supplementation may interfere with the metabolism of oral hormones like estrogen and oral contraceptives. Individuals at risk for hormone-sensitive conditions should avoid red clover. A typical dose reducing hot flashes ranges from 40 to 160 milligrams daily.

Soy isoflavones: Isoflavones are plant compounds found in the legume family (for example, kudzu, fava bean, chick pea, soybean) that act as phytoestrogens and may have anticancer activity. Supplemental use of soy isoflavones, particularly genistein, may be helpful for reducing menopausal complaints: daily doses of 35 to 120 milligrams have been used for this purpose. Side effects include gastrointestinal upset and headaches. The cautions listed under red clover apply to soy isoflavones. Individuals who are sensitive or allergic to soy should avoid this supplement.

Gut Support

A key word for the sacral chakra is "balance." Just as the different fats have to be kept in harmony in the body, so too do the different microorganisms living in our gut. Seeding the lower gut with healthy bacteria is essential for keeping the gut lining healthy and free of microorganism overgrowth. These bacteria need to be fed with prebiotics, or special fibers, to keep them active and producing healthful substances for the colon. Agents that engage the sacral chakra in its peristaltic dance can be helpful for releasing stuck energy and allowing stagnated energy to move forward and out.

Many individuals appear to have lower gut complaints, and the psycho-spiritual-energetic origins of these issues could be very diverse. However, no matter where the issues stem from, they are in some way linked to the ability to let go—whether that means expanding into to one's creativity, emotions, or relationships, or releasing any aspects of these things that do not serve the body or soul. Utilize the healing element of water in the form of baths, steam rooms, or additional hydration to enable the body to expand and release emotions and old thought patterns.

Probiotics *(Lactobacilli, Bifidobacteria)***:** Supplementation with beneficial microorganisms, such as the many strains of *Lactobacilli (L. acidophilus, L. amylovorus, L. brevis, L. bulgaricus, L. casei, L. crispatus, L. delbrueckii, L. fermentum, L. lactis, L. plantarum, L. reuteri, L. rhamnosus, L. salivarius, L. helveticus, L. paracasei)* and *Bifidobacteria (B. bifidum, B. breve, B. infantis, B. lactis, B. longum)* found in yogurt, is essential for keeping the intestinal tract and immune system healthy. Without adequate amounts of probiotics, the structure of the intestine may degrade, leading to reduced gut immunity and impaired gut movement (peristalsis). Cramping, bloating, loose or constipated stools, and fatigue may result. Oral therapy with various combinations or doses of these bacteria has been used for acute diarrhea, bacterial overgrowth, atopic dermatitis, immune dysfunction, candidiasis, irritable bowel syndrome (IBS), and ulcerative colitis. When the number of beneficial bacteria is more than the number that are detrimental, we can more easily remain in a state of health (and sacral chakra balance). If you are taking antibiotics, take your probiotic supplement at least a couple of hours afterwards.

Prebiotics: In order for healthy bacteria to thrive in the gut, they need to feed on specific substrates. Prebiotics are long chains of sugars from fruit and vegetable sources (for example, asparagus, Jerusalem artichokes, onions, chicory root, and leeks) that are not able to be broken down by the body's digestive enzymes, but can be metabolized by bacteria that live in the colon. Two common supplemental sources of prebiotics include fructo-oligosaccharides (FOS) and inulin. Since prebiotics fuel the growth of specific bacteria in the gut, they can work in tandem with probiotics. A typical daily dose is 4 to 10 grams. Note that higher doses exceeding 8 to 10 grams daily may result in gas, bloating, and abdominal pain due to the intestinal bacteria fermentation. Start supplementing very gradually with small amounts, building up to your gut tolerance level.

Aloe vera *(Aloe barbadensis)***:** When taken internally, pure aloe vera liquid can soothe the gastrointestinal tract and help to relieve inflammation in the body. It can also help the bowels move, releasing stuck energy in the sacral chakra. Take care not to use aloe vera liquid on an ongoing basis because you can develop an intolerance to its effects. Be cautious when taking it together with supplements or drugs that lower blood glucose, act as a diuretic, or have laxative effects.

Additional Individual Supplements

Inositol: *See the third eye chakra chapter for specific details.* Supplementation with inositol (4 grams plus 400 micrograms folic acid per day) has been used to affect fertility by improving ovarian function in women, particularly those with polycystic ovary disease.

Beta-carotene: Beta-carotene is an orange pigment that belongs to the family of red, orange, and yellow pigments known as carotenoids. It is found concentrated in fruits and vegetables such as carrots, sweet potatoes, apricots, peaches, and spinach. Due to its orange color, this carotenoid resonates with the orange vibration of the sacral chakra. From a physiological perspective, most of the ingested beta-carotene from foods or supplements converts to vitamin A in the body. The remainder of beta-carotene collects in the skin, adrenals, and corpus luteum. There is no daily recommended amount, but deficiency may be associated with increased cell damage by free radicals and a weak immune system. Excessive intake can lead to a yellow-orange color of the skin, particularly the palms of the hands and soles of the feet. Beta-carotene supplements are not to be taken by the general population, and, specifically, smokers should not supplement with beta-carotene.

The sacral chakra embraces the idea of opposites, which is another reason why beta-carotene links to this center: like other antioxidants, it has the ability to function in a dual manner, either as a protective antioxidant or as a potentially harmful pro-oxidant, depending on its environment. Studies have shown that some populations, like smokers and those exposed to high levels of asbestos, do not benefit from beta-carotene supplementation.

CHAPTER 6

SUPPLEMENTS FOR POWER AND TRANSFORMATION (SOLAR PLEXUS CHAKRA)

Our worst fear is not that we are inadequate, our deepest fear is that we are powerful beyond measure.
NELSON MANDELA

CHAKRA DESCRIPTION

With the anchor of the root chakra and the flow of the sacral chakra, we are now ready for action and exchange with the outside world. The solar plexus chakra fuels the body by taking in raw materials from the outside—as food, supplements, or even thoughts, beliefs, and opinions—sifting them through the body and energetic system, extracting what is needed, and transforming the raw material into the energy of action. This chakra gives us the ability to distill and transform energy so that we can respond in the manner we feel most aligns with our identity. It is also the seat of the raw intellect, a repository of the fleeting thoughts, conversation exchanges, and internal dialogue. These streams of information become further processed in the higher chakras, like the heart and third eye chakras, to become part of the landscape of one's internal wisdom.

Words associated with the solar plexus chakra: *alchemy, beliefs, distillation, exchange, ego, fire, identity, inspiration, logic, manifestation, power, presence, self-esteem, transformation, yellow.*

CHAKRA ANATOMY AND PHYSIOLOGY

The solar plexus chakra embodies the fire element and stimulates transformation on many levels. The digestive organs represent the dynamic nature of this chakra, which serves as a filter and combustion chamber that harnesses energy for the cells of the organism.

Solar plexus chakra anatomy: Gallbladder, liver, pancreas, small intestine, stomach.

HEALTHY INDICATIONS

A person who is comfortable with her powerful, confident self is someone who expresses the needs of the self, manifests personal power in the world, integrates perceptions from the outer world with internal beliefs and opinions, thinks logically, creates harmony between their internal and external worlds, and is able to be decisive and firm when confronted with choices.

UNHEALTHY INDICATIONS

If you answer yes to a majority of the following questions, your solar plexus chakra may need healing:

- *Do you feel stressed from the responsibilities of life?* Do situations, no matter how small or large, seem to tax your internal reserves? Is your life drained of any sweetness and filled with burdens? Are you tired all the time and remain unsatisfied after eating? When the solar plexus is burned out, there is a drain on the entire being—a drain that prevents the chakra from interacting with the outside world and that manifests as stress or fatigue. Eating becomes erratic, and the appetite insatiable due to the lack of fulfillment from daily experience. Life feels like drudgery when we are empty of energy.

- *Are you overweight, particularly in the abdomen?* Do you suffer from digestive complaints like indigestion, acid reflux, or bloating? When there is excessive, unprocessed energy in the solar plexus chakra, we may take on physical symptoms of this excess, such as too much belly fat, too much acid, too much gas, and too much undigested food.

- *Do you lack confidence in your ability to succeed in the world, or are you overly egotistical?* Do you analyze your achievements to the extent that you discount them or inflate them to excessive proportions? Are you a perfectionist or obsessive with details? Are you driven to the point of excess, believing that you can do everything on your own and actually trying to "do it all"? The solar plexus chakra is an action-oriented aspect to the individual, but sometimes this ambition and motivation shift into high gear and overdrive—clearly an unhealthy, unbalanced state that ultimately leads to exhaustion and the "never enough" syndrome (no object, event, or accomplishment is satisfying).

SUPPLEMENTS FOR THE SOLAR PLEXUS CHAKRA

MACRONUTRIENTS AND MACRONUTRIENT SUPPLEMENTS

Carbohydrate

Carbohydrate, the fuel for the solar plexus chakra, comes in a variety of forms, including quick and simple or slow and complex. The needs of the solar plexus chakra and its corresponding physiology determine the most nourishing form. For a majority of us, the solar plexus chakra is on constant overdrive—we are continually burning the candle at both ends. In this instance, it is best to choose carbohydrate sources of the slow and complex of variety for a long, continued supply of energy. An example of this type of carbohydrate is soluble fiber. In supplement form, bulk soluble powders made from psyllium seed, guar gum, and fruit pectin are available. They work to clear the intestines of toxins and soften the stool. The action of these soluble fibers comes from their capacity to swell and become gummy when eaten (which is why they need to be consumed quickly after being mixed with water). The viscous mass they become in the gut is good, because like a net, it traps many things within it. Including soluble fiber with a meal helps slow the release of sugar into the blood, thus helping balance blood sugar, which is a prime solar plexus function. In the lower part of the gut, in the neighborhood of the sacral chakra, soluble fibers can be fermented by bacteria, creating nutrients like short-chain fatty acids, which keep the colon healthy.

VITAMINS

Biotin

Description and Sources: A water-soluble vitamin found in brewer's yeast, cooked eggs, meat, milk, and whole grains.

Functions: Metabolizes carbohydrate, protein, and fat. Facilitates cell growth, fatty-acid production, B-vitamin utilization, healthy hair, skin, and nails.

Intake: Biotin needs may be increased in people on renal dialysis, smokers, and in those with hair loss and brittle nails. There is some question as to whether biotin requirements are increased during pregnancy.

Deficiency: Anemia; depression; hair loss; scaly rash; lethargy; impaired utilization of glucose, which leads to increased blood sugar; muscle pain; soreness of tongue; and nausea. Deficiency can result from consumption of raw egg whites for an extended period (weeks to years); cooking egg white denatures the protein that prevents absorption of dietary biotin.

Overuse: Not known to be toxic.

Interactions: Use of antiseizure medications (carbamazepine, phenobarbital, phenytoin, etc.) is associated with lower biotin levels in the body. Antibiotics can alter the normal bacteria in the gut that make biotin; therefore, it may be worthwhile to take a biotin supplement concurrent with antibiotics. Biotin supplementation may increase the effects of medications or supplements that lower lipids in the blood. High supplemental vitamin B5 (pantothenic acid) can result in decreased biotin absorption in the gut.

Relationship to Chakras: Primary chakra: solar plexus. Secondary chakras: root, crown. Through its effects on metabolism, biotin resonates with the solar plexus. It also gives its energy to the root chakra for cell growth and maintenance of healthy protein structures and supports the crown chakra through its role in nerve function.

Vitamin B1 (thiamin)

Description and Sources: A water-soluble vitamin in whole grains, legumes, meats (particularly liver), egg yolks, vegetables, and fruit.

Functions: An important nutrient for carbohydrate metabolism. Eating high amounts of carbohydrate increases the need for thiamin. Also essential for nervous system activity, brain function, and cognition.

Intake: May be important to supplement those with mental illnesses, cardiovascular disease (for example, congestive heart failure), and nerve problems (for example, paralysis, nerve pain).

Deficiency: People consuming a diet high in refined carbohydrates or high in alcohol are susceptible to thiamin deficiency. Deficiency manifests as a condition referred to as beriberi, which includes neurological symptoms such as nerve pain, exaggerated reflexes, and diminished sensation in hands and arms (dry beriberi), or cardiovascular symptoms such as rapid heart rate, an enlarged heart, and breathing difficulties (wet beriberi). Deficiency may also cause brain abnormalities.

Overuse: Relatively uncommon.

Interactions: Consumption of large amounts of coffee and tea can convert thiamin into a form that cannot be used by the body. This reaction can be prevented with adequate intake of vitamin C or by ingesting sufficient thiamin. Raw fish or shellfish contain an enzyme that degrades thiamin. Cooking inactivates this enzyme.

Relationship to Chakras: Primary chakra: solar plexus. Secondary chakras: third eye, crown. Thiamin resonates most with the solar plexus chakra because of its specificity for carbohydrate (the fuel for the solar plexus chakra) metabolism. It allows for the extraction of energy from carbohydrates. Without it, we cannot hold the life force that comes through us, and as a result, we become prone to the development of neurological and cardiac symptoms (crown and heart chakras). Thiamin also relates to the third eye and crown chakras directly through its role in brain and nervous system function.

Vitamin B2 (riboflavin)

Description and Sources: A water-soluble vitamin found in cheese, egg yolks, fish, legumes, meats, and milk.

Functions: Assists in metabolism of carbohydrate, fat, and protein through its role in cellular respiration, or harnessing energy from macronutrients. Riboflavin is also needed for red blood cell formation, antibody production, and the metabolism of tryptophan. It may be useful in carpal tunnel syndrome.

Intake: Heavy exercisers and those under stress may need more riboflavin. Daily doses under 10 milligrams are thought to be beneficial for those at risk of riboflavin deficiency. Taking 200 to 400 milligrams per day may reduce the frequency of headaches or migraines. Lower doses of 2.6 milligrams daily could be helpful for preventing cataracts.

Deficiency: Cracks or sores at the corners of the mouth, dermatitis, hair loss, light sensitivity, decreased mental response, eye disorders. Strenuous exercise may increase the body's need for riboflavin.

Overuse: No direct toxic effects in humans, but very high doses may lead to cataract formation, retinal diseases, and diarrhea. Can also cause a yellow-orange discoloration in urine.

Interactions: May improve iron utilization.

Relationship to Chakras: Primary chakra: solar plexus. Secondary chakra: root. Like its sister B vitamins, riboflavin helps the solar plexus chakra to maintain a steady energy exchange. It also plays a role in root chakra activities that promote grounding, such as building the red blood cells and immune cells.

Vitamin B3 (niacin, niacinamide, nicotinic acid)

Description and Sources: A water-soluble vitamin found in beef liver, brewer's yeast, vegetables, dairy products, whole grains, red fish (tuna, salmon), coffee, and tea.

Functions: Used for the metabolism of carbohydrate, fat, and protein (called oxidation-reduction reactions) and for the synthesis of the body's energy currency, ATP. The niacin and nicotinic acid forms reduce cholesterol (see the heart chakra chapter). Niacin can be synthesized from the amino acid tryptophan if sufficient vitamin B6, riboflavin, and iron are available.

Intake: In people with abnormal levels of blood fats (high triglycerides, low HDL-cholesterol, high LDL-cholesterol), 1,200 to 3,000 milligrams of niacin has been used.

Deficiency: Severe niacin deficiency results in a condition called pellagra, or a constellation of symptoms that includes a thick, scaly rash, a bright tongue, vomiting, diarrhea, depression, headache, memory loss, and, if left untreated, ultimately death.

Overuse: Too much nicotinic acid can result in a facial flush, sometimes experienced with a painful, tingling sensation, after ingestion. Niacinamide ingestion does not cause facial flushing. Ingestion of high amounts of either nicotinic acid or niacinamide could lead to nausea, vomiting, liver damage, and may decrease the action of insulin, resulting in an impairment of the body's ability to use glucose.

Interactions: Avoid alcohol when taking supplements. Taking large amounts of niacin could aggravate gout. Exercise caution if taking with statins, due to potential heightened risk of muscle soreness (called myopathy).

Relationship to Chakras: Primary chakra: solar plexus. Secondary chakra: heart. All vitamins contribute to the energy body; however, this vitamin has a particularly heavy contribution. Since vitamin B3 is directly involved in metabolism reactions and is required for making the classic energy currency that the body recognizes as ATP, it has an integral role in the solar plexus chakra. It is truly a powerhouse energy supplement for our physical and spiritual bodies. Its influence is so strong that it impacts the heart chakra through its potent effects on blood vessels.

Vitamin B5 (pantothenic acid, calcium pantothenate)

Description and Sources: A water-soluble vitamin found throughout the food supply. Its name is derived from the Greek word "pantothen," meaning "from everywhere."

Functions: Essential for the metabolism of carbohydrate, protein, and fat and for the function of the adrenal gland and production of adrenal hormones.

Intake: Individuals with allergies, or with fatigue, or who eat high amounts of refined foods may need additional pantothenic acid (25 to 100 milligrams daily has been recommended as a minimum dose by nutritional experts). For those who experience chronic stress, 100 to 500 milligrams daily has been recommended as a therapeutic dose. Diabetes and alcoholism may lead to deficiency of this vitamin.

Deficiency: Relatively rare perhaps due to the ubiquity of pantothenic acid in foods, but can manifest as fatigue, headache, nausea, tingling in hands and feet, muscle weakness in legs, gastrointestinal complaints, and increased susceptibility to infections.

Overuse: Not typical, but can result in diarrhea.

Interactions: Individuals taking oral contraceptives may have increased need for pantothenic acid.

Relationship to Chakras: Primary chakra: solar plexus. Secondary chakra: root. Pantothenic acid is a core vitamin for the energetic wiring and functioning of the solar plexus chakra due to its role in the metabolism of all the macronutrients. Additionally, it assists the root chakra in its fight-or-flight response by supporting the energy of the adrenal gland and the manufacture of adrenal hormones.

Vitamin B6 (pyridoxine)

Description and Sources: A water-soluble vitamin found in a wide variety of foods, including cereal grains, beans, animal foods like meat and eggs, and some fruits and vegetables.

Functions: As part of the entire B vitamin family, vitamin B6 plays a role in metabolism of macronutrients, especially protein. On its own, it is integral to forming hemoglobin, the protein in the blood that carries oxygen; to keeping the heart healthy through its reduction of the damaging amino acid product homocysteine; and in assisting in the synthesis and metabolism of neurotransmitters like serotonin and dopamine.

Intake: Individuals taking antidepressants or oral contraceptives may have an increased need for pyridoxine: supplementation with 25 to 50 milligrams daily (not more than 100 milligrams due to toxicity) might be helpful. PMS symptoms may be reduced if taking 50 to 100 milligrams pyridoxine daily. Alcoholism tends to significantly lower vitamin B6 levels in the body.

Deficiency: Dermatitis, sore tongue (glossitis), depression, confusion, convulsions, anemia.

Overuse: Doses over 100 milligrams daily are not advised due to the potential to cause changes in nerve function. Other indications of overuse include nausea, vomiting, loss of appetite, abdominal pain, and headache.

Interactions: May interfere with the effects of some drugs, particularly those that impact the brain and nervous system. Women on oral contraceptives may have lower levels of pyridoxine. Use of isoniazid (a drug used to treat tuberculosis) may result in vitamin B6 deficiency.

Relationship to Chakras: Primary chakra: solar plexus. Secondary chakras: root, sacral, heart, third eye, crown. Vitamin B6 integrates the top and bottom chakras because it assists the solar plexus with metabolism, especially the metabolism of protein. Its resonance with protein connects it to the root chakra, and its association with neurotransmitters and brain function connect it with the third eye chakra; thus, it unites these two energy centers. Vitamin B6 also works with its sister B vitamins folic acid and B12 to reduce the toxic amino acid homocysteine and thus keep the energy circulating freely in the heart chakra. Finally, vitamin B6 is closely tied to central nervous system function, for which the crown chakra provides the energetic underpinning.

Vitamin B12

See the root chakra chapter for specific details. In addition to its many associations with the root chakra, vitamin B12 is required in the metabolism of fat and carbohydrate under the direction of the solar plexus chakra. A particular protein, called intrinsic factor, needs to be present in the stomach for vitamin B12 to be absorbed into the body. Therefore, a healthy functioning stomach (and solar plexus chakra) is essential for adequate body levels of vitamin B12.

B-vitamin complex

The entire B complex comprises eight water-soluble vitamins: thiamin (B1), riboflavin (B2), niacin (B3), pantothenic acid (B5), pyridoxine (B6), biotin (B7), folic acid (B9), and cyanocobalamin (B12). Although each of them has individual functions, they also work together in the solar plexus chakra, helping produce energy from carbohydrates, proteins, and fats. This chakra requires a network of nutritional and energetic support since it is the body's main entrance and exit for energy. Because of its incessant activity, it is difficult to keep balanced, and solar plexus chakra imbalances and deficiencies (evidenced by the rise in metabolism disturbances such as obesity and type 2 diabetes) are prevalent in our society. Therefore, it is reasonable that this chakra would require a vibrational support team.

MINERALS

Chromium

Description and Sources: A trace element in a wide variety of foods, including grains, seafood, beef, and dairy products like cheese.

Functions: Chromium plays a pivotal role in the metabolism of macronutrients, particularly carbohydrate, and is used for improving the body's ability to dispose of glucose (sugar).

Intake: Supplementation is often advocated for those with diabetes and conditions associated with blood-sugar imbalance, such as hypoglycemia, decreased energy, and polycystic ovary disease. Recommended dose for those with type 2 diabetes is 200 to 1,000 micrograms, divided throughout the day. Newer research shows reduced food intake and cravings in overweight women taking 1,000 micrograms chromium versus a placebo.

Deficiency: May occur with stress, malnutrition, and pregnancy. Diabetics may have lower body chromium levels. Symptoms include poor glucose control, nerve dysfunction, and weight loss.

Overuse: Weight gain, cognitive and nerve dysfunction, headaches, sleep disturbances, mood changes, vomiting, kidney damage.

Interactions: Chromium competes with iron and zinc for absorption and transport; take them separately. If taking chromium supplements together with insulin, hypoglycemia may result. Do not take thyroid medication (such as Synthroid) at the same time as a chromium supplement—take them separately (for example, take a chromium supplement three to four hours after taking Synthroid).

Relationship to Chakras: Primary chakra: solar plexus. Chromium has a unique resonance with the solar plexus chakra. It lends an energetic hand to this chakra by allowing energy in the form of glucose to be efficiently delivered and received by the whole body, especially by the main metabolic workhorses like the liver and muscle. Chromium helps an imbalanced solar plexus chakra to regain its robust nature.

BOTANICALS/OTHER

Blood-Sugar Support

The simplest energy currency of the solar plexus chakra is glucose. When glucose balance is thrown off in the body, it signifies that the energy of the solar plexus chakra is imbalanced. The body's inability to use glucose effectively spills over into other physiological effects and, as a result, other chakras. For example, extended periods of dysglycemia (abnormal levels of glucose in the blood) will lead to changes in the blood vessels and blood circulation (heart chakra), altered appetite (throat chakra), difficulty concentrating and focusing (third eye chakra), and nervous system dysfunction like nerve pain in the outer extremities (crown chakra). So regulating blood-glucose levels in the solar plexus chakra is essential for maintaining the balance of all the energy centers.

When blood-sugar balance is an issue, the questions to ponder may include: Where am I squandering my resources? Why am I not finding sweetness in my life? What are some things I can do or what opinions, beliefs, and thoughts can I let go of in order to make life more enjoyable? Energy imbalance in the body, from a physical or spiritual perspective, can be detrimental to the functioning of the entire organism.

Alpha-lipoic acid: A potent antioxidant that aids in carbohydrate metabolism. At 600 to 1,200 milligrams daily, it has been used to improve tissues' sensitivity to insulin in diabetics. Helps regenerate antioxidants like vitamins C and E. Used extensively to reduce symptoms of diabetic nerve pain (diabetic neuropathy; see the crown chakra chapter). Nausea and skin rash have been reported with its use. If alpha-lipoic acid is used in conjunction with other blood sugar-lowering agents (for example, chromium), there can be a dramatic lowering effect on blood sugar, so precaution should be taken.

Cinnamon *(Cassia cinnamon):* Although the data are conflicting, cassia cinnamon might favorably impact glucose and insulin levels. In diabetes,

1 to 6 g daily (1 teaspoon equals 4.75 g) has been used. Large amounts may be toxic to the liver. Do not use in conjunction with supplements or drugs that have hypoglycemic or hepatotoxic effects.

Bitter melon, bitter gourd *(Momordica charantia):* Bitter melon, a vegetable commonly eaten in Asian countries, can lower blood glucose. A number of active compounds in bitter melon influence insulin action. May be taken as a very bitter fresh juice (50 to 100 milliliters daily), as a dry powder (3 to 15 grams daily), or as a standardized extract (100 to 200 milligrams three times daily). Excessive intake can lead to diarrhea, gastrointestinal upset, and stomach pain. Taking bitter melon with other herbs or supplements that reduce blood sugar can cause even more blood-sugar lowering (possibly to the point of hypoglycemia, or when the blood sugar has dropped below the normal range) than if taken alone. Not recommended for use in pregnancy.

Fenugreek *(Trigonella foenum-graecum):* Fenugreek seeds, possibly due to their soluble fiber content, have been shown to decrease blood-sugar levels in diabetics when 15 grams of the seeds (soaked in water) were taken daily, or when the seeds were taken in the form of an extract (1 gram daily). Fats in the blood may also be reduced with fenugreek supplementation, although further research is necessary. Side effects include allergic reactions, gastrointestinal complaints, and hypoglycemia when the seeds are in large doses. Exercise caution when using together with supplements or drugs that have anticoagulant or hypoglycemic actions. Do not use if you are pregnant or lactating. Not to be taken by children.

Gymnema *(Gymnema sylvestre):* The leaf of this woody shrub, which is native to India and Africa, has been used for thousands of years in India to treat "honey urine" (diabetes). A 400 milligrams extract of gymnema, taken daily by diabetics, reduces blood sugar. It is thought that gymnema works by decreasing the uptake of sugar in the intestines and also by stimulating the beta-cells in the pancreas (these cells produce insulin). Use caution if taking it together with blood-sugar-lowering supplements or drugs.

Ginseng (American ginseng; *Panax quinquefolius):* The ginseng root is an ancient tonic used to restore energy and combat fatigue. It helps to reduce the amount of stress hormones that congest the solar plexus chakra, thereby helping hormones to work more effectively. Taking 3 grams before a meal can lower blood glucose in diabetics. Do not confuse American ginseng with Siberian or Panax (Asian) ginseng. Side effects include gastrointestinal complaints, insomnia, and agitation (especially in schizophrenics). May increase the effect of supplements or drugs with hypoglycemic activity. Do not take together with monoamine oxidase (MAO) inhibitors or with warfarin. Since some ginseng extracts have estrogenic effects, anyone with a history of or with active hormone-sensitive cancers should avoid these extracts.

Digestive Support

Over time, with aging and perhaps under stressful conditions, the ability of the solar plexus chakra to extract energy from foods might become impaired. The breakdown of foods starts within the throat chakra, in the mouth, which produces amylase in saliva to degrade starch. If we do not chew our food adequately and give careful attention to what we put into our mouths, it may be more difficult to digest and assimilate these substances in the solar plexus chakra region. Various supplements, such as digestive enzymes, can be used to assist in the process. If we continue to eat foods without being able to digest them in the mouth, stomach, and intestines, we may not receive the nourishment we need to deal with our daily events—a condition adding to the stress in the solar plexus. Additionally, as the undigested food makes its way through the intestine and encounters a leaky gut (sacral chakra), large food particles (seen by the body as invaders) may be taken up in the blood, ultimately causing an immune reaction (root chakra). Consequently, a fine-tuned digestive process, spearheaded by a healthy solar plexus chakra, can prevent the effects of poor digestion on the lower chakras.

When digestive disorders arise, it may be appropriate to reflect on this question: what am I unable to assimilate or "digest"?

Digestive enzymes (amylases, lipases, proteases): Commercial enzyme preparations made from animal or fungal sources are available. These supplements often combine three types of enzymes—proteases, amylases, and lipases—which assist in the breakdown of the three main macronutrients: protein (proteases), carbohydrate (amylases), and fat (lipases). Bromelain is an example of an enzyme derived from pineapple that may help to digest protein. In addition to bromelain aiding in protein digestion, some preliminary studies have demonstrated that it may reduce pain in those with osteoarthritis, knee pain, and muscle pain. Do not take bromelain in conjunction with other anticoagulants as bleeding and bruising may result. Bromelain supplementation may increase the activity of oral antibiotics—take them separately. Since they work directly on ingested food, they should be taken with a meal. Do not drink large amounts of water during mealtimes, as this may dilute the enzyme concentration and impair their activity.

Hydrochloric acid: With aging commonly comes a lack of significant stomach acid to digest dietary protein. Supplemental hydrochloric acid (for example, in the form of betaine hydrochloric acid, or betaine HCl) can be taken with meals to assist the stomach in this process. (See the "Macronutrients" section of the root chakra chapter for more details.)

Stomach Support

The first organ of transformation within the solar plexus chakra area is the stomach. With too much incoming energy that cannot be effectively processed, the stomach may become overheated, inflamed, acidic, and unable to digest. Potent yellow botanicals, like turmeric and ginger, can provide the stomach with the vibration it needs to cool down and move energy through the body.

Ginger root *(Zingiber officinale):* The yellowish ginger root has been traditionally used to treat stomach upset, nausea, vomiting, and morning sickness. Although it has a reputation of being a protective for the stomach, it can cause stomach distress, like heartburn, abdominal pain, or diarrhea, if taken in large amounts. Ginger has also been used to reduce inflammation, thin the blood, and lower cholesterol. Due to its blood-thinning properties, it is not recommended for those who take anticoagulants. Additionally, individuals who have gallstones should avoid it, since it has stimulating effects on bile secretion. One of ginger's most common applications is for morning sickness: 250 milligrams four times daily or 500 milligrams twice daily have been used. For healthy stomach movement, 1,000 to 1,200 milligrams ginger has been studied. Extended use during pregnancy is not advised.

Turmeric *(Curcuma longa):* This root, commonly used as a seasoning and as a constituent of curry powder, has been shown to exhibit strong antioxidant and anti-inflammatory properties. In various studies, taking a total of 2000 milligrams (500 milligrams four times daily) or 3000 milligrams (600 milligrams five times daily) has been shown to reduce dyspepsia symptoms. The major active compounds are the curcuminoids. Side effects may include nausea and diarrhea. Use caution if taking it together with anticoagulant supplements or drugs.

Liver Support

The liver is very consistent with the mission of the solar plexus chakra: it employs detoxifying enzymes to filter what out what the body does not need. This process occurs through two sequential steps: first, toxins are converted into water-soluble compounds. Second, a chemical group, like a sulfur-containing compound, is added to assist in the toxins' release from the body. For this reason, our ability to clear metabolic clutter comes from the power of the liver. In addition to being one of the major organs of detoxification, the liver is the central site for processing of fat after a meal: after we eat, the fats from the meal travel from the digestive system and can be subsequently found in the blood in a protein-containing compound. The last stop is typically the liver. Too many fatty foods, too many highly processed foods full of sugar, or too much alcohol may cause congestion in the liver. Various nutritional approaches can support this precious organ, and assist in its ability to detoxify body poisons and to route and dispose of fats in the body in the best way.

Liver issues such as fat accumulation, inflammation, or toxicity might require you to examine the efficient function and energetics of the liver. What is preventing you from action? What toxicity, either from the environment or from within (emotions, thought patterns), is causing you to become stuck and inflamed?

Choline: Choline used to be considered a B vitamin until it was discovered that it could be produced in the liver. Dietary sources include egg yolks, liver, meats, nuts, and wheat germ. The actions of choline are not limited to the terrain of the solar plexus, although much of its function radiates from this hub. Choline assists in gallbladder regulation and prevents liver dysfunction. Because choline plays a role in fat and cholesterol metabolism, choline deficiency can lead to fatty liver (known as hepatic steatosis). The heart chakra benefits from choline because choline donates special chemical groups (methyl groups) to reactions that reduce levels of homocysteine, a harmful amino acid that has been connected with heart disease. The third eye chakra benefits from choline because choline is a building block for acetylcholine, the neurotransmitter responsible for memory and mood. In choline deficiency, brain function and memory are impaired. Finally, choline is required for the transmission of nerve impulses from the brain through the central nervous system (overseen by the crown chakra). Side effects of choline supplementation include profuse sweating, fishy body odor, gastrointestinal complaints, and vomiting.

Dandelion root *(Taraxacum officinale):* The bright yellow dandelion plant has been used traditionally for liver complaints, as a diuretic, and to stimulate appetite. It may have some impact on the digestive process through its ability to increase bile production. Dandelion should not be taken in conjunction with prescription diuretics, or by those with biliary tract obstruction or gallstones. It may also alter how certain drugs are metabolized, so check with your healthcare professional if you are taking medications. In some individuals, it may cause allergic reactions.

Milk thistle (silymarin, *Silybum marianum):* The seeds of the milk thistle contain the potent active silymarin, which is particularly effective for liver disorders. It prevents toxins from infiltrating liver cells, stimulates new liver-cell growth, and may possess anti-inflammatory, immune-enhancing properties that are particularly beneficial in liver conditions. It may help decrease insulin resistance, reduce dyspepsia, and protect against kidney damage. It is generally well tolerated, but allergic reactions and gastrointestinal effects, like laxation, may be experienced. Milk thistle supplements may alter the metabolism of specific drugs like warfarin and diazepam. The plant extract (not necessarily the seed) may have estrogenic effects; therefore, individuals with hormone-sensitive conditions should avoid it. Individuals with an iron-storage disease (hemachromatosis) should avoid taking milk thistle. Different preparations and doses have been used: for hepatic cirrhosis, 420 milligrams of a milk thistle extract containing 70 to 80 percent silymarin, and for chronic active hepatitis.

Metabolism Support

The bulk of B vitamins are instrumental for metabolizing carbohydrate, protein, and fat, typically by playing a role in core processes such as cellular respiration or in oxidation-reduction reactions. There are other actives that may work together with these vitamins to move the energy through the solar plexus chakra. You will read in chapter 8 that the throat chakra is also connected to the body's metabolism through the thyroid gland, which sets the metabolic tone for the whole person. Try to apply the solar plexus chakra's connection with fire to the concept of the metabolic fire: How do we burn fuel (nutrients) for energy? If metabolism is slow, what in our life needs igniting or catalytic action?

L-carnitine: L-carnitine, a compound related to the structure of amino acids and derived from animal foods, assists in transporting long-chain fats into the mitochondria (powerhouse of the cell) so that these fats can be burned for energy. The human body can make L-carnitine if it has sufficient iron, thiamin, vitamin B6, vitamin C, and the amino acids lysine and methionine. When needed, L-carnitine can convert in the body to acetyl-L-carnitine (see the crown chakra chapter). Low levels in the body can lead to mental confusion, heart pain, muscle weakness, and obesity. Supplementation may be useful in conditions where fat metabolism is impaired. Conditions involving fatigue, like chronic fatigue syndrome and autoimmune diseases, may most benefit. Side effects include gastrointestinal disturbances, fishy body odor, and seizures. Do not supplement with L-carnitine if you are taking thyroid hormone or supplements or drugs that have anticoagulant properties. The dose for combating fatigue related to a clinical condition is 2 grams daily.

Green tea extract: Green tea extracts, rich in the polyphenol epigallocatechin gallate (EGCG), can increase fat and calorie burning along with suppressing appetite. The individual constituents in green tea, including caffeine and catechins, may be responsible for these effects. Side effects include gastrointestinal complaints, agitation, dizziness, insomnia, tremors, confusion, and liver toxicity (particularly when a specific ethanolic extract of green tea is taken). Exercise caution when taking green tea extract in conjunction with supplements or drugs that have anticoagulant activity. Physiological reactions due to caffeine may be enhanced if green tea extract (nondecaffeinated) is taken together with other caffeine-containing products. Green tea reduces the absorption of iron from plant sources and may decrease the activity of folic acid. Do not use it together with supplements or drugs that have stimulatory effects on the central nervous system. A recent study showed that a supplement containing a green-tea extract composed of 890 milligrams polyphenols and about 366 milligrams of EGCG led to increased fat burning and improved insulin sensitivity in healthy humans compared with a placebo. Similarly, overweight men, taking 300 milligrams of EGCG for just two days, experienced more fat burning than when they were taking a placebo.

CHAPTER 7

SUPPLEMENTS FOR LOVE AND COMPASSION (HEART CHAKRA)

Love makes your soul crawl out from its hiding place.
ZORA NEALE HURSTON

CHAKRA DESCRIPTION

Of all the aspects of an individual, the heart center, as a conduit to love and healing, is probably the most widely recognized. The heart chakra territory is the meeting place where body and spirit come together in equal parts and radiate out to others in the acts of giving and receiving. Joy, contentment, and gratitude are the fruits of the heart chakra. In this space, an individual can choose to accept and give love in equal measure. When the heart chakra opens to love, its energy extends out several feet and blossoms like a rose. The power of love can pour forward through the heart chakra to act as a healing salve for yourself, others, and the web of life.

Words associated with the heart chakra: *air, compassion, depth, devotion, emotional wisdom, empathy, forgiveness, giving, gratitude, green, joy, kindness, love, loyalty, receiving.*

CHAKRA ANATOMY AND PHYSIOLOGY

The heart chakra allows our being to express and unfold through the circulation of breath and blood. The intricacy of the heart pump and lung branches moves these vital substances throughout the body. When we are full of these vital forces and they are flowing freely, healing love can move through us. Love extends out through the arms and fingers when we warmly embrace someone, hold hands, or give and receive.

Heart chakra anatomy: Armpits, arms, blood vessels, breasts, hands, heart, lungs, lymphatic system, shoulders, wrists.

HEALTHY INDICATIONS

A person who is comfortable with their loving self is someone who expresses love; gives thanks to self, others, and God; sees love as the underlying foundation for everything they do; loves the self and others; constructs healthy boundaries regarding feelings and their expression; and balances giving and receiving.

UNHEALTHY INDICATIONS

If you answer yes to a majority of the following questions, your heart chakra may need healing:

- *Do you feel that you either overgive to others or overreceive from others?* Do you feel it is difficult to say no to others, and are you resentful when you haven't said no? Does overnurturing lead you to feel exhausted and bitter? Keeping the heart chakra in balance through a healthy mix of receiving and giving is essential. Often, overgiving is encouraged in the Western culture, and it can be depleting in the long term. Giving the heart chakra permission to receive can be liberating and, in the end, allows us to be better at giving to others, whether we give words of wisdom or acts of service.
- *Do you suffer from heart disease, chest pains, or breathing difficulties?* Do you have difficulty eating a healthy diet or taking care of yourself? Constriction and lack of energy flow in the heart chakra region can

contribute to heart and circulatory problems. Heart disease is the number one killer in the United States. What in the American society is causing this restriction and pain in the heart? What is the collective heart bound by? Stress, lack of passion, lack of love?

- *Do you feel that you are unable to process your emotions in a way that is healthy for you and others around you?* Do you take on others' emotions? Have you had emotional wounds that have impaired your ability to give and receive love? Are you unable to forgive others? A wounded heart chakra is one that sees life as full of sadness and grief. Being closed off from our deepest feelings results in feeling numb about life. These individuals are not able to cry or to touch and be touched by others.

SUPPLEMENTS FOR THE HEART CHAKRA

MACRONUTRIENTS AND MACRONUTRIENT SUPPLEMENTS

L-arginine: This amino acid from animal foods may be helpful in cardiovascular conditions, such as coronary heart failure, angina (chest pain), and high blood pressure, along with blood-vessel impairments, like erectile dysfunction. L-arginine is converted into a compound (nitric oxide) that allows the blood vessel to dilate, or expand. Side effects include abdominal pain and bloating, diarrhea, and gout. Do not combine L-arginine with supplements or drugs that lower blood pressure or that work by opening blood vessels. For congestive heart failure, 6 to 20 grams has been given in three divided doses per day. For high blood pressure, 6 grams daily has been used therapeutically (in combination with other nutrients).

Soy protein: Soy protein, derived from the green soybean (edamame), nourishes the heart chakra, mainly due to its ability to lower blood fats and blood pressure (particularly diastolic blood pressure) and prevent cardiovascular disease. For lowering blood fats, 20 to 50 grams of soy protein daily is recommended. Soy protein is unique because it contains all the amino acids necessary to support growth; therefore, it is one of the few vegetable proteins that can be efficiently used by the body. In addition to being a nutritionally complete protein, it contains an array of other heart chakra actives, including (1) **phytoestrogens** (isoflavones, lignans), or weak, estrogenlike compounds, (2) **phytosterols** (plant sterols, plant stanols), or compounds that resemble the structure of cholesterol, and, as a result, are able to block the absorption of dietary cholesterol in the gut, and (3) minerals.

Besides its effects on blood fats, soy protein also has the potential to influence other heart chakra organs, including the breasts. Population studies with Asian women indicate that a diet high in soy foods results in a reduced risk for breast cancer; however, studies of the North American population are lacking. More research is needed to understand the impact dietary soy and soy supplements might have on breast cancer. It has been suggested that women with breast cancer or a history of breast cancer reduce or avoid soy intake because knowledge of its effects is lacking.

The lower chakras (root and sacral) are linked to the actions of soy. Soy protein, particularly due to its isoflavone content, may reduce hot flashes and the overall severity of menopausal symptoms. Consumption may also increase bone mineral density by enhancing bone formation and reducing bone breakdown.

Side effects include gastrointestinal upset, such as changes in bowel pattern (constipation, diarrhea), bloating, and nausea. Soy is a major allergen. Individuals who are allergic to soy should avoid consuming it. In individuals with iodine deficiency, soy may inhibit thyroid-hormone synthesis. It has the potential to interact with monoamine oxidase (MAO) inhibitors, oral estrogens, tamoxifen, and anticoagulant drugs.

VITAMINS

Vitamin B3

See the solar plexus chakra chapter for specific details. One of niacin's primary uses is reducing high blood fats like LDL cholesterol (the "bad" cholesterol) and triglycerides, and increasing HDL cholesterol (the "good" cholesterol). Since high doses of niacin (1,200 to 3,000 milligrams per day) are usually needed to affect cholesterol, it is found not only in dietary supplement form, but also as a prescription drug. Niacin is often taken in combination with statins (prescription drugs to lower cholesterol); however, this should be done only under the

supervision of a qualified healthcare professional, because niacin can potentially worsen the side effects of statins. The main side effect with high doses of
niacin (not niacinamide) is flushing in the face, neck, and chest, which suggests
an increase in the amount of energy rushing into the heart chakra space.

Vitamin B6

See the solar plexus chakra chapter for specific details. Vitamin B6 (100 milligrams
daily, taken after eating) works together with folic acid to reduce levels of the
blood vessel-damaging compound homocysteine by about one-third.

Vitamin K (phylloquinone, vitamin K1, menaquinone, MK-7, vitamin K2)

Description and Sources: The vitamin K family consists of a group of
fat-soluble compounds. The two members that have special relevance to human nutrition are vitamin K1 (also known as phylloquinone) and vitamin K2
(menaquinone, MK-7). Vitamin K1 is found primarily in plant sources such
as leafy green vegetables (e.g., broccoli and spinach) and vegetable oils (e.g.,
soybean oil), while vitamin K2 is obtained from animal foods like meat,
cheese, and eggs, and also from fermented foods (for example, natto, a fermented soy food that is popular in Japan, contains high levels of vitamin K2)
since it is made by bacteria.

    Functions: Required for normal blood clotting and for a healthy bone
structure.

    Intake: Postmenopausal women, who are particularly vulnerable to
bone loss, may benefit from a vitamin K supplement. When postmenopausal
women with low bone mineral density took 5 milligrams of vitamin K1 for
two to four years, they experienced fewer bone fractures than women who
did not take a supplement. Healthy young children had improved levels of a
modified bone protein (which is good for bone health) when they were given
a vitamin K2 supplement (45 micrograms daily for eight weeks) compared
with those children given placebo. Additionally, individuals with cardiovascular disease may experience delayed progression of plaque buildup, as
demonstrated in a study using 500 micrograms of vitamin K1 daily for three
years.

Deficiency: Excessive bleeding due to abnormal blood clotting (for example, nosebleeds, bleeding gums, heavy menstrual bleeding). Individuals with fat malabsorption disorders such as Crohn's disease or cystic fibrosis may have lowered absorption of vitamin K by the gut. Taking certain medications, such as antibiotics, may result in vitamin K deficiency.

Overuse: No known toxicity with high doses.

Interactions: Vitamin E reduces the absorption of vitamin K and can alter its activity in the body. Vitamin K may reduce the activity of anticoagulant medications like warfarin (Coumadin).

Relationship to Chakras: Primary chakra: heart. Secondary chakra: root. Vitamin K has a dual nature that allows it to service both the heart and root chakras. By playing an essential role in normal blood coagulation, such as in case of a wound or injury where the skin is broken and bleeds, vitamin K allows the heart chakra to establish boundaries to prevent its energy from flowing endlessly. From an energetic perspective, this function is crucial to balancing the cycle of receiving and giving in those who tend to give too much. Its connection to boundaries extends down to the root chakra, because it is able to support the proteins that compose the bone matrix.

MINERALS

Iodine

See throat chakra chapter for specific details. Iodine supplementation (80 micrograms per kilogram body weight of molecular iodine) has been used for fibrocystic breast disease. The breast tissue concentrates iodine to a greater extent than the thyroid gland. In animal studies, iodine deficiency alters the function of mammary glands. Women with breast cancer have lower iodine levels in their breast tissue compared to women without cancer or women with benign fibroadenoma. Breast cancer rates are lower in populations that eat diets high in iodine, such as in Japan, than they are in populations eating less iodine. The relationship between dietary iodine and iodine supplementation and breast cancer continues to be investigated.

Magnesium

Description and Sources: A silver-white alkaline metal within the earth's crust and in a wide variety of foods, such as legumes, grains, vegetables, seeds, nuts, dairy products, meats, and chocolate.

Functions: Used for the activity of hundreds of enzymes in the body. The skeleton is a depository of magnesium, but it can also be found in the fluid in which cells are bathed, where it facilitates cellular reactions.

Intake: Many people are deficient in magnesium because of lack of intake or due to conditions that may deplete the body's magnesium reserves. The following puts one at risk for developing magnesium deficiency: alcoholism, chronic stress, renal disorders, malabsorption syndromes (for example, Crohn's disease, celiac disease, gastric bypass surgery or other intestinal surgery), diabetes, and taking medications (diuretics, antibiotics, chemotherapy). Diabetics may benefit from 300 to 400 milligrams of magnesium per day. Individuals with restless leg syndrome may have low magnesium—consider supplementation if levels are lower than normal. Doses of 450 to 1,000 milligrams daily have been used for reducing high blood pressure, 600 milligrams daily for preventing migraines, 150 to 750 milligrams daily for osteoporosis prevention, and 200 to 360 milligrams daily for reducing PMS symptoms.

Deficiency: Confusion, insomnia, gastrointestinal issues, abnormal heart rhythms and spasms, diabetes, loss of appetite, weakness, chronic pain, numbness, and fatigue.

Overuse: Very similar to symptoms of deficiency—diarrhea, loss of appetite, low blood pressure, difficulty breathing, nausea, vomiting, muscle weakness, heart irregularities.

Interactions: High doses of calcium or zinc can decrease magnesium absorption; it is best to take them separately. Several medications can interact with magnesium supplements and also alter magnesium levels in the body. If you are taking any medications, check with your healthcare practitioner before taking magnesium.

Relationship to Chakras: Primary chakra: heart. Secondary chakras: root, sacral, solar plexus, throat, third eye, crown. Magnesium is the protectorate of the heart and the blood vessels, providing this network with an environment that enables the heart to take in energy and beat regularly. It gives the heart in the necessary vibrational and electrical energy to keep it wired to life force. In addition to bathing the cells in the body (connecting it to the sacral chakra), it also stabilizes the skeleton. The balance between magnesium and calcium, or the bond between the heart and root chakras, is essential for living out our heart's mission. Magnesium feeds the sacral chakra waters by maintaining the proper pH for many reactions to occur within the extracellular space. Several of the enzymes that harness energy from foods require magnesium, and therefore, the solar plexus is impacted by magnesium. Small amounts of magnesium can invigorate throat chakra energy by restoring hearing lost to excessive noise. And finally, magnesium is connected to the third eye and crown chakras through its influence on neurotransmitter function and the nervous system. Magnesium is one of the few substances that feeds the entire energetic circuit.

Potassium

Description and Sources: A silvery white alkaline compound found in wide variety of fruits and vegetables.

Functions: Maintains electrical properties of cells, which impact the function of cardiac, smooth, and skeletal muscle, as well as brain and nerve function.

Intake: Supplementation may help reduce high blood pressure and risk of stroke and cardiovascular disease.

Deficiency: Skin problems (severe dryness, acne), changes in gastrointestinal function (constipation, diarrhea), heart-rhythm irregularities, blood-pressure dysfunction, muscle weakness and fatigue, nausea, vomiting. A number of medications can result in low potassium in the body.

Overuse: Stomach upset, nausea, weakness, low blood pressure, heart problems.

Interactions: Using potassium with blood-pressure or other medications that retain potassium in the body may lead to high potassium levels.

Relationship to Chakras: Primary chakra: heart. Secondary chakras: third eye, crown. Potassium carries the energy of fruits and vegetables, which feeds the heart chakra. Together with other minerals, like calcium and magnesium, potassium can ensure that the heart receives and gives out sufficient energy. Additionally, it provides a conduit through which the brain and nerves can be connected to higher energetic vibrations.

BOTANICALS/OTHER

Blood-Lipid Support

The heart organ and web of blood vessels that extend out from it are sensitive to the amount of lipids (fats) flowing through the circulating blood. Too much of certain types of fats combined with the effects of high blood pressure can stress the blood vessels, ultimately leading to injury and plaque buildup. Over the long term, the blood-vessel walls narrow, and circulation is reduced. There is an increased risk of blocked arteries and blood clots that can impede blood flow to the heart, causing a heart attack. By keeping blood-cholesterol levels low, the heart chakra energy can remain active and moving. Sacral and heart chakras can fulfill their unified mission of balancing fats in the body when we complement a diet of foods low in long-chain saturated fats and trans fats (sacral chakra) with nutritional supplements that help the heart chakra stay unblocked. When the circulatory network is congested by fats, ask the following questions of the heart: What is causing blocks in my ability to love life? Within my heart, what is accumulating that no longer serves me?

Phytosterols (plant sterols, plant stanols, beta-sitosterol): Compounds derived from plant oils, like vegetable or soybean oils, look like cholesterol, but actually block the absorption of cholesterol in the intestine. Some food products, like margarines and breakfast cereals, have added phytosterols and advertise the U.S. Food and Drug Administration (FDA) claim that phytosterols help reduce cholesterol. There are two types of phytosterols: plant sterol esters and plant stanol esters. Both are present naturally in plant foods like fruits, vegetables, and vegetable oils. At least 1.3 grams of plant sterol esters or 3.4 grams of plant stanol esters daily, along with a low-fat (particularly saturated fat), low-cholesterol diet, are recommended for heart health. Overall, these compounds are well tolerated, although in some individuals, they can cause nausea and gastrointestinal upset. There has been concern that phytosterols can lower absorption of fat-soluble vitamins like vitamin E and carotenoids such as beta-carotene. Individuals with a rare disease known as sitosterolemia should avoid phytosterols.

Red yeast rice *(Monascus purpureus):* This nutritional product is the end result of rice fermented with *Monascus purpureus* yeast. The fermentation process produces a number of cholesterol-lowering actives, one of which is lovastatin (a drug prescribed for cholesterol reduction). Therefore, red-yeast-rice supplements work in a way similar to that of statin drugs, inhibiting the enzyme that manufactures cholesterol in the body. If not fermented correctly, the rice can become contaminated with citrinin, a toxin that causes kidney failure. Side effects include those also associated with statin drugs, such as liver damage, elevated liver enzymes, and muscle weakness. Red yeast rice may lower the body's levels of coenzyme Q10 and affect the metabolism of botanical supplements like St. John's wort. Other effects may include gastrointestinal complaints, dizziness, and allergic reactions. This supplement may interact with several drugs; use it only under the supervision of a qualified healthcare professional. A dose of 2.4 grams daily has been used, but cholesterol-lowering effects may occur with lower doses (1.2 grams per day).

Circulation Support

The river of blood moving through the veins is important for the delivery of oxygen and nutrients to the rest of the body. Without healthy flowing blood, stagnation can result in various parts of the body and contribute to blocks in other chakras. For example, when blood collects in the legs due to weak capillaries, we become stagnant within not only the heart chakra, but also the root chakra. If we have poor circulation to the brain, we may not get the materials we need for better thinking, memory, and concentration. The flow of blood in the body is an indirect indication of the flow of energy in and from the heart chakra.

Bilberry fruit extract *(Vaccinium myrtillus):* See third eye chakra chapter for more details. The fruit and leaf of this blueberry relative has a high concentration of the purple pigments anthocyanidins, which help maintain the integrity of the capillaries. They may also lower blood glucose, which can help to heal rifts between the heart and solar plexus chakras. Anthocyanidins' role in eye health also connects this supplement to the third eye chakra. This extract may interact with hypoglycemic supplements and drugs, ultimately requiring that doses of antidiabetic drugs, like insulin, be adjusted. Consult a qualified healthcare provider if you wish to supplement with bilberry and you are diabetic.

Bioflavonoids: The term *bioflavonoids* refers to thousands of individual plant compounds commonly found in fruit, especially citrus fruits. Typical bioflavonoids in dietary supplements are quercetin, hesperidin, and rutin. Together with vitamin C, they work to strengthen the capillaries and veins and to promote healthy blood circulation. Note that bioflavonoids from grapefruit may interfere with the metabolism of certain drugs. Side effects of quercetin supplementation include headache, a tingling sensation in the extremities, and kidney toxicity, while those of rutin include headache, flushing, rashes, or gastrointestinal discomfort. Commonly recommended quercetin dosages are 400 to 500 milligrams three times per day. A daily dose of 730 milligrams for twenty-eight days reduced blood pressure in people with high blood pressure. Individuals with vein and blood circulation disorders (chronic venous insufficiency) who took 2 grams of rutin per day for five years had reduced swelling.

Garlic: Even though garlic as a food feeds the root and solar plexus chakras through its pungent properties, the essence of supplemental garlic vibrationally impacts the heart chakra to the greatest extent. Garlic extracts are known for their ability to lower blood pressure and blood fats and to reduce blood clots, thus opening up the energetic circulation of the heart chakra area. Doses between 600 and 1,200 milligrams daily may produce these beneficial effects. Side effects may include offensive breath and body odor, gastrointestinal discomfort, nausea, and vomiting. Exercise caution if using garlic supplements while taking other supplements or medications that have anticoagulant effects. Supplemental garlic interacts with the metabolism of a number of medications; consult your healthcare professional before taking it. Note that the odorless garlic preparations may not contain the active compound, allicin.

Gotu kola *(Centella asiatica):* Gotu kola has a number of effects on the body, and the strongest evidence suggests it restores blood circulation. A gotu kola extract (120 to 180 milligrams daily) has been shown to improve circulation and decrease swelling in individuals with venous insufficiency. It may cause gastrointestinal complaints, nausea, drowsiness, and liver toxicity (elevated liver enzymes). Do not use with herbs, supplements, or drugs that affect the liver or that have sedative properties.

Grape seed extract: Grape products, particularly grape seed extract, are abundant in compounds that, through their antioxidant action, help improve chronic venous insufficiency, vein health and vasodilation (blood-vessel opening). These products also have decrease the ability of a blood clot to form, which is needed for keeping the blood flow unobstructed through the blood vessels, a key factor in preventing a stroke or heart attack. Side effects include headache, gastrointestinal complaints, cough, and sore throat. Grape seed extract may interact with anticoagulant supplements or drugs or those that lower blood pressure. A higher starting dose (75 to 300 milligrams) for the first couple of weeks, followed by a lower dose (40 to 80 milligrams daily) for the longer term, has been suggested for vein health.

Horse chestnut *(Aesculus hippocastanum):* The seeds of this plant are most commonly used in the treatment of chronic venous insufficiency. Side effects include dizziness, nausea, headache, itching, gastrointestinal upset, and kidney damage. It may cause allergic reactions in some people. It also may interact with supplements or drugs that have anticoagulant or hypoglycemic (blood-sugar-lowering) effects. For chronic venous insufficiency, a dose of standardized extract containing 50 milligrams of the active (aescin) is taken twice daily.

Additional Individual Supplements
Coenzyme Q10 (CoQ10, ubiquinone): A fat-soluble, vitaminlike substance found in all cells in the body, especially in the heart, liver, kidney, and pancreas. It functions as an antioxidant, plays a role in energy production, aids blood circulation, and helps stimulate immune function. It also lowers blood pressure and strengthens heart muscle. Even though the body can produce coenzyme Q10 in small amounts, these levels are not always adequate. Statins, drugs used for cholesterol reduction, are known to reduce blood levels of coenzyme Q10. Supplementation in the range of 100 to 200 milligrams daily, in two to three separate doses, has been used for a variety of conditions, including heart health.

Green food powders (alfalfa, barley grass, broccoli powder, chlorella, chlorophyll, spirulina, wheat grass): Green food powders carry the vibratory frequency of the color green, which is very cleansing and healing for the heart chakra. Foods like alfalfa, spirulina, and young grasses (wheat grass, for example) supply an optimal ratio of nutritious, bioavailable compounds, including chlorophyll, amino acids, enzymes, and minerals such as calcium, magnesium, and potassium. The cumulative vibration of these constituents captures the complexity of the primordial essence from which life originated. Chlorophyll is especially helpful in cleansing the blood. Eating these green food powders is like pushing an internal reset button, bringing us back to our heart's mission: to love.

Hawthorn *(Crataegus laevigata):* The leaf, fruit, and flower of this plant have been used for several aspects of heart function, including reducing cholesterol and the symptoms of heart failure, which in turn strengthens the heart muscle and heart rhythm. For people with heart failure, a dose of 900 to 1,800 milligrams of a standardized extract has led to beneficial effects. Side effects include vertigo, dizziness, gastrointestinal complaints, fatigue, rash, palpitations, headache, and agitation. Hawthorn may interact with supplements and drugs that affect blood pressure or blood-vessel dilation.

Lycopene: An association may exist between dietary consumption of this red-colored pigment (found in high amounts in cooked tomatoes [applying heat to the tomato makes the lycopene more available] and other red fruits and vegetables) and the risk of cardiovascular disease. Women consuming at least seven servings per week of tomato-based products had a 30 percent reduction in cardiovascular disease risk. Additionally, higher concentrations of lycopene in the blood have been correlated with a decreased risk of cardiovascular disease in women. Lycopene may also nourish another heart chakra organ, the lungs. Daily supplementation with 30 milligrams lycopene for one week resulted in significant protection against exercise-induced asthma. The root chakra is also nourished by lycopene, particularly through its actions on the prostate gland (see the chapter on the root chakra for details).

CHAPTER 8

SUPPLEMENTS FOR COMMUNICATION AND TRUTH (THROAT CHAKRA)

Self-expression must pass into
communication for its fulfillment.
PEARL S. BUCK

CHAKRA DESCRIPTION

As we climb the chakra tree, we realize the skills that allow us to take in and synthesize the complexity of life. Up from the heart chakra is situated an energetic nexus (referred to as the throat chakra) where a multitude of body functions (breathing, chewing, drinking, eating, hearing, laughing, smelling, swallowing, talking, tasting, yawning) are synchronized and respond to the outside world. On a higher level, we can coordinate the diversity of tasks we are capable of in order to express our truth, creativity, and authenticity. The throat chakra enables harmony of the whole self by communicating the internal world to the external one, primarily through the vehicle of sound. This chakra serves as the conduit, or birth canal, through which emotions, thoughts, and passions are freed from the lower chakras—from sacral to heart chakras—and expressed in a true, honest manner. When the throat chakra is open and clear, a person is released from the shackles of fear and can more fully surrender to their path, as their spirit intends them to be.

Words associated with the throat chakra: *aquamarine, authenticity, choice, communication, coordination, Divine will, expression, faith, freedom, senses, sound, speech, surrender, truth, voice.*

CHAKRA ANATOMY AND PHYSIOLOGY

There is much physiological activity in the realm of the throat chakra. In many ways, it begins the transformative process of receiving information from the outside and bringing it inside, as well as allowing each person's internal voice to make its way outward. Through its oversight of the senses of hearing, tasting, and smelling, it experiences the environment, and its perceptions meet the inner landscape. These experiences assist the individual in knowing what is true for them. The exchange is complete when the voice tells the external world what that truth encompasses.

Throat chakra anatomy: cheeks, chin, ears, larynx, lips, mouth, neck, nose, pharynx, throat, thyroid gland, tongue, upper esophagus.

HEALTHY INDICATIONS

A person who is comfortable with their authentic self is someone who releases control and accepts life, speaks their truth, expresses themselves through their voice; acknowledges a higher spiritual presence, accepts their life path, and learns through their sensory experience.

UNHEALTHY INDICATIONS

If you answer yes to a majority of the following questions, your throat chakra may need healing:

- *Do you feel inhibited or overly open when communicating with your voice?* The voice is a conduit of personal expression and creativity. Do you have a tendency to talk too much, trying to fill the silence or dodge important issues related to communication? Or are you silent because of lack of connection with your stream of creativity? How we use our voice says volumes about the throat chakra. When imbalanced, it may be shut down, resulting in a suffocating feeling. Or it may be too excessive and open to the extent that there is nothing that gets held back, making words as sharp as razors or turning them into garbled nonsense. If we are cut off from our wellspring of creativity, our throat chakra will become desiccated and the voice will become raspy.

- *Are you afraid to surrender your will to a higher power—to embrace choice and, at the same time, know that a perfect life design has been laid out before you?* Do you find it difficult to pray or to have faith in yourself, others, or a spiritual force? Constriction and control are signs of a disharmonious throat chakra. When we become overly absolute and confined to a certain way that we want to live our lives, we cut ourselves off to the abundance of opportunities and wisdom that may help us to live more authentically. Being humble allows us to step into true leadership and grace.

- *How do you coordinate all of the activity in the throat chakra area, including breathing, talking, swallowing, chewing, smelling, and hearing?* Are any of these limited (meaning not doing it at all) or chaotic (perhaps engaging in more than one of these at once)? How do you synthesize and integrate one or more of them with each other? We are wired to receive much sensory information, but without a clear throat chakra, our breathing may become erratic, eating can become mindless and excessive, talking can become rambling, and smelling and hearing can become painfully heightened or deadened. Looking at how we work with our senses and how we engage the throat chakra portal of entry for the body on many levels can provide us with insight as to how we live. For example, if you consistently find yourself talking while trying to chew food, are you also trying to process life while trying to express yourself? If you find yourself prone to shallow breathing, is there something about life that you are unwilling to take in?

- *Are you gulping in the experience of life at a speed that does not allow information to be integrated into your personal perception of truth?* A throat chakra with excessive energy will burn up energy so quickly that you feel dissatisfied and longing for more; physically it manifests as high metabolism. On the other hand, a throat chakra deficient in energy will translate into a feeling that you are plodding through life at an extremely sluggish pace, feeling disengaged from all those around you. It may manifest physically as a slow metabolism or a state of not being able to process and integrate energy into your own.

SUPPLEMENTS FOR THE THROAT CHAKRA

Deciding whether to take supplements: The throat chakra governs choice. Do you actively choose to take supplements, or do you allow others—the media, vendors, and other individuals—to make that selection for you? To decide if taking supplemental forms of nutrients is beneficial for your energy physiology, tune into your subtle-body wisdom through your chakras for your ultimate answer. Work with a healthcare professional for clarity and focus. Reflect on your process, journal about it, meditate, and pray to know what nutrients, if any, would serve your highest good.

Consciousness when taking supplements: Swallowing a pill or chugging down a spoonful of liquid is easy for some individuals, and, as a result, taking dietary supplements may become automatic or routine. I have seen many people simply toss a handful of pills down their throat without taking time to ingest them as though they were the powerful substances they truly are. These people often have lives full of chaos and they see supplements as one of the "band-aids" to keeping them well; however, there is meaning in not only what supplements we take, but how we choose to take them in. The throat chakra asks us to ingest all substances mindfully. In the same way that chewing food thoroughly balances the throat chakra, being fully present and communicating your intention for taking the dietary supplement will assist the body and spirit in integrating the vibratory message carried in the dietary supplement.

Forms of supplements: Dietary supplements and botanicals come in a variety of forms, including tablets, capsules, liquids, softgels, chewables, and powders. The throat chakra welcomes an array of media. It may not always be practical (or easy) to swallow large tablets. Sometimes certain nutrients are more available to the body in liquid form. Eating a chewable may allow the nutrient to be absorbed within the mouth cavity. Allow your throat chakra the flexibility of choice, and refrain from becoming wedded to any single delivery system.

Supplement variety: The throat chakra feeds on variety and enjoys being presented with choices in all forms. Taking in the same supplements each day can cause the body to become programmed, almost putting it on automatic pilot. I often advise that people practice tuning into their own body (and throat chakra) by asking their inner selves what is needed day by day rather than moving through the motions of taking lots of supplements without thought. Some people come in for a consultation with their bags of dietary supplements and, when asked, they don't even know why they are taking them. We become so used to simply adopting other people's opinions that we lose sight of our own body's truth.

In fact, my personal belief based on my clinical experience is that it may be worthwhile to change your supplement routine regularly so that the body does not become too energetically attached to any particular dietary supplement. Getting just the right dose for a defined period of time, rather than in endless duration, may help the body immediately shift into the vibration needed for healing. If we are constantly confronted with a vibration from a supplement, it may lose its initial healing charge. I have heard from various people who begin taking certain supplements, find they work for awhile, and then after some time, they don't notice any effect. It is though the body "acclimates" to the energy of the supplement, and if there are no other changes that are made in a person's life other than taking the supplement, it makes good sense that the body would return to its original dysfunctional pattern. *Thus, keep in mind that a dietary supplement's purpose is to equip you with the energy you need to make a shift—it will not make the shift automatically without you supporting it on a conscious level.* Additionally, there are some supplements that are clearly not meant to be taken long-term, like some of the plants such as andrographis and echinacea for enhancing immune function. Taking high amounts of supplements like vitamin C for extended periods of time and then not taking them may compromise body functions and even result in deficiency-like symptoms. This effect may be due to the body rewiring its activity with a certain level of a supplement on a regular basis. When the large amounts have dwindled, the body has to shuffle its physiology to meet a new baseline of activity. Practice listening to your body's needs or work with your healthcare professional to alternate or rotate your supplements.

MACRONUTRIENTS AND MACRONUTRIENT SUPPLEMENTS

Soy protein: Even though soy protein is beneficial for cardiovascular disease (see the chapter on the heart chakra), it may reduce the production of thyroid hormone in individuals who have thyroid problems, and especially those who have iodine deficiency (see the iodine listing under "Minerals," below). Those with iodine deficiency and thyroid issues should limit their consumption of soy.

VITAMINS

Vitamin A (retinol): *See the root chakra chapter for specific details.* Vitamin A deficiency can occur together with iodine deficiency and lead to impaired thyroid function. In studies with children who are iodine and vitamin A deficient, vitamin A supplementation helped the body to use iodine from iodized salt.

Vitamin D: *See the root chakra chapter for specific details.* The four parathyroid glands are nestled next to the thyroid gland, yet they do not have the same function as the thyroid gland. Their job is to ensure that there is an adequate level of calcium in the body. To accomplish this task, they release parathyroid hormone to help activate vitamin D in the body so it can stimulate calcium absorption in the gut. The parathyroid glands will start making more of their hormone if vitamin D levels are too low, causing a condition called hyperparathyroidism. If you are deficient in vitamin D (your healthcare practitioner can do a lab test), supplementation may be worthwhile.

MINERALS

Iodine
Description and Sources: An essential nutrient found in foods grown in soil or harvested from the sea, or in foods with added iodine, like iodized salt.

Functions: Iodine concentrates in the thyroid gland and is used to make iodine-rich hormones that control many physiological processes, like metabolism.

Intake: Individuals with fibrocystic breast disease may be helped by supplementing with iodine. It has been recommended not supplementing with more than 600 micrograms of iodine per day because of the ability of high levels of iodine to inhibit thyroid hormone synthesis.

Deficiency: Iodine deficiency has serious effects on brain development and is associated with mental retardation. The classic deficiency symptom is a goiter, or an enlarged thyroid gland.

Overuse: Too much iodine results in a burning sensation in the mouth and throat, sore teeth and gums, a metallic taste in the mouth, and gastric upset, to name a few symptoms.

Interactions: Discuss iodine supplementation with a healthcare practitioner if you are taking thyroid medications.

Relationship to Chakras: Primary chakra: throat. Secondary chakra: heart. Proper iodine levels are necessary for the health of the throat chakra. With too little, the throat chakra becomes sluggish, unable to support the workings of the organs it oversees, like the thyroid gland. With too much, the throat chakra goes on overdrive, dispersing and losing energy to the outside. The effects of iodine deficiency in the throat chakra can extend energetically to the heart chakra. Too little iodine can result in energy stagnation in the heart chakra, which can eventually manifest as fibrocystic breast disease.

Selenium

See the sacral chakra chapter for specific details. The thyroid gland has the highest concentration of selenium in the body, as this mineral is needed for the manufacture and metabolism of thyroid hormones. Specifically, it is a cofactor for the enzyme that converts one thyroid hormone (T4, thyroxine) into another (T3, triiodothyronine)—a reaction that does not happen efficiently in hypothyroidism. In the case of iodine deficiency, selenium deficiency can worsen hypothyroidism. Taking 200 micrograms selenium daily has been shown to reduce blood levels of a marker (called antithyroid peroxidase) of autoimmune thyroiditis.

Thyroid Gland Support

The thyroid gland, nestled in the throat chakra vicinity, is one of the main points controlling metabolism. Whereas the solar plexus chakra contains the organs of transformation and energy exchange, the throat chakra provides the energetic framework and coordinates the secretion of hormones for those processes to occur, and it determines how the entire body (not just the digestive organs) will integrate the energy. When excessive energy comes into this gland (hyperthyroidism), the throat chakra will attempt to quickly integrate the energy, but it may be dissipated into symptoms such as an accelerated heart rate, breathlessness, and nervousness. When not enough energy comes into the thyroid gland (hypothyroidism), it will have difficulty keeping up with the body-wide assimilation of information. As a result, the movement of energy through the body tissues will be slow. An individual with low thyroid function may feel tired, depressed, and cold, and their skin, hair, and nail quality will decline.

Sea kelp (bladderwrack, *Fucus vesiculosus*): Because of their ability to merge dual elements, namely water and earth, sea plants resonate with the integration and coordination functions of the throat chakra. Specifically, sea plants such as brown seaweed *(Fucus vesiculosus)* nourish the throat chakra due to their iodine content. Note that sea plants are also prone to having heavy concentrations of metals found in the sea, such as cadmium and arsenic. Excessive intakes of sea kelp, because of its iodine content, can lead to thyroid imbalances (similar to the effects of iodine). Consult with a healthcare practitioner before taking sea kelp with medications for the thyroid gland or anticoagulant drugs.

Throat Support

The throat is a vessel through which the lower chakras, particularly the heart chakra, can express their essence—the survival needs of the root chakra, the emotions and creativity of the sacral chakra, the power and ego of the solar plexus, and the love and compassion of the heart. It allows for breath to be inhaled and exhaled, for food to be swallowed and accepted, and for the voice to form and exit. When we are troubled by expressing certain thoughts, feelings, or opinions, the throat may become dry, and even develop into a sore throat or tonsilitis, especially if we are inflamed about something. Unsaid truths may manifest as polyps or other growths in this area. It is important to keep the throat moist and lubricated for the flow of expression that is meant to occur.

Licorice *(Glycyrrhiza glabra):* Licorice has a number of properties that make it desirable to take for a sore throat. In addition to its ability to help clear mucus, it can also soothe and coat the throat. For a sore throat, it can be prepared as a tea by steeping 1 teaspoon of licorice root in hot water for two to three minutes, or a slice of raw licorice can be sucked on. Do not use licorice during pregnancy. Taking an excessive amount over an extended duration (several weeks) can lead to changes in sodium and fluid levels, electrolyte imbalance, and elevations in blood pressure. Avoid using with antihypertensives, anticoagulants, corticosteroids, and estrogens. May have estrogenic effects; do not take if hormone-sensitive condition is present.

Marshmallow *(Althaea officinalis):* The root and leaf of the marshmallow plant have been used as a traditional remedy for sore throat. Like slippery elm, it contains mucilages (or long chains of sugars combined with protein) to coat the throat and help suppress cough. It is typically prepared as a tea, using either the dried leaf or dried root. Not to be taken by pregnant or lactating women. May reduce blood sugar and, as a diuretic, lead to increased urination. Use caution when using marshmallow with supplements or drugs that lower blood sugar or those that may be affected by increased urination. Take marshmallow root or leaf separately from medications, as it is known to impair drug absorption in the gut.

Slippery elm *(Ulmus rubra):* The inner bark rind from this North American deciduous tree contains mucilages that, when taken orally, provide a soothing film over mucous membranes, like those in the throat. Slippery elm is often taken in the form of lozenges and used for sore throats and coughs. Pregnant and lactating women should avoid it.

Sinus Support and Allergies

Conditions like allergies involve both the root and throat chakras. Allergic rhinitis (often called nasal allergies or hay fever) is a specific expression of the allergy category. Since the root chakra oversees immune system function, allergies actually start within this chakra, and the symptoms blossom within the throat chakra, since the latter provides a direct opening to the outside. When the immune system becomes overactive due to environmental substances like animal dander, dust, mold, or plant pollen, the throat chakra region is affected with an array of symptoms, such as coughing; headache; itchy nose, throat, mouth, skin, and eyes; runny nose; inability to smell; sneezing; sore throat; and wheezing. Allergic sinusitis calls us to examine what we are overreacting to in our environment.

Blue-green algae *(Spirulina platensis):* Spirulina, a complex mixture of single-celled organisms from the sea, contains a variety of nutrients, including protein, B vitamins, fat, and minerals. It has been shown to stimulate immune function and reduce the symptoms of allergic reactions. Taking a specific spirulina supplement at 2 grams daily for twelve weeks led to a reduction of an inflammatory marker (interleukin-4) in individuals with allergic rhinitis. Ensure that the supplement is free of toxic blue-green species contaminants. These contaminants can produce liver-toxic substances that can result in death. Do not take if you have an autoimmune disease or take immunosuppressants. Side effects include gastrointestinal complaints.

Butterbur *(Petasites hybridus):* The leaf, rhizome, and root of butterbur may be useful in reducing symptoms of allergic rhinitis. Specific butterbur extracts that do not contain naturally occuring toxic compounds called pyrrolizidine alkaloids have been shown to improve nasal symptoms. Butterbur appears to lower compounds related to the immune response (such as histamines and leukotrienes) in the blood of individuals with allergic rhinitis. It may also be effective for migraines. Side effects include belching, headaches, itchy eyes, diarrhea, asthma, and fatigue. Some individuals may be allergic to this plant family. Taking butterbur may influence the metabolism of certain drugs. Confirm that the extract is free of alkaloids. Specific butterbur extracts are available for short-term use for relief of allergic rhinitis symptoms.

Methylsulfonylmethane (MSM): One study of fifty people with allergic rhinitis showed that taking 2,600 milligrams of MSM for thirty days resulted in decreased respiratory symptoms. *See the root chakra chapter for more details on MSM.*

Quercetin and Bromelain: *See the heart chakra chapter for additional effects of quercetin.* Quercetin supplementation at 250 to 600 milligrams three times daily, taken five to ten minutes before meals, may be helpful for calming the inflammatory-immune response to allergies. It has been suggested that quercetin may work more effectively if taken together with the pineapple enzyme bromelain (400 to 500 milligrams three times daily of an 1,800 to 2,000 m.c.u. potency bromelain). As a side note, bromelain is highly resonant with the solar plexus chakra because of its ability to break down and transform food as an enzyme. Side effects of bromelain include allergic reactions in those with pineapple allergy and gastrointestinal disturbances. Exercise caution if using bromelain with other supplements or drugs that have anticoagulant effects. Zinc may inhibit the activity of bromelain; take them separately.

Stinging nettle *(Urtica dioca):* The above-ground parts of the stinging nettle plant have been traditionally used for allergies and allergic rhinitis. This supplement appears to work best when taken at the first start of symptoms. It may be beneficial because of its quercetin content. Quercetin has anti-inflammatory effects and dampens the release of histamine from immune cells. Side effects include gastrointestinal complaints, sweating, and allergic skin reactions. May interact with supplements or drugs that have effects on blood pressure, blood sugar, central-nervous-system depression, fluid excretion, and coagulation. Typical dose for allergic rhinitis is 300 milligrams three times daily.

Common Cold

Whereas allergies are due to a hyperactive immune system, a common cold can result when immune defenses are low and a viral invader is present. Like allergies, the common cold is connected to the root and throat chakras. Supplements discussed in the root chakra chapter for supporting immune function, particularly vitamin C, zinc, and echinacea, would assist the throat chakra in combating cold symptoms.

Jaw Support

Temporomandibular joint (TMJ) problems manifest as tightness and constriction in the jaw muscles and indicate a restriction and excessive buildup of energy in the throat chakra. TMJ issues may evolve into an inflammatory condition like osteoarthritis (see the root chakra chapter). With TMJ osteoarthritis, nutritional supplementation for joint support might be helpful. If you have TMJ issues, ask yourself, what am I not saying? Instead of vocalizing your thoughts, you might feel more comfortable expressing them in some other way, like journaling, singing, or developing a personal mantra that can support you.

Glucosamine sulfate: In a study with people with TMJ osteoarthritis, glucosamine sulfate, at 500 milligrams taken three times daily, was found to be more effective than ibuprofen for reducing pain.

Sensory Support

The throat chakra provides us with a gateway to the external world through the senses of hearing, smelling, and tasting. If any of these senses are not functioning properly, examine whether there is an energy block keeping you from in taking in more of the surroundings or experiencing and interacting with life.

Magnesium: *See the heart chakra chapter for specific details.* As demonstrated in human and animal studies, magnesium supplementation, even at low doses, may prevent noise-induced hearing loss.

Zinc: *See the root chakra chapter for specific details.* Zinc supplementation (25 to 100 milligrams) may help with taste dysfunction (a condition called hypogeusia) in people who have low zinc levels. It may also improve taste in those with various taste disorders stemming from medications, radiation, and trauma.

CHAPTER 9

SUPPLEMENTS FOR INTUITION AND IMAGINATION (THIRD EYE CHAKRA)

*The more and more each is impelled by that
which is intuitive, or the relying upon the soul force within,
the greater, the farther, the deeper, the broader,
the more constructive may be the result.*
EDGAR CAYCE

CHAKRA DESCRIPTION

Although most people might deny it, everyone has access to intuition. The third eye chakra represents the intuitive part of a person, providing a path to one's internal wisdom and to spiritual guidance. Since it oversees not only the intuition, but also the faculties of the mind, spanning the continuum from logic to imagination, it can be accessed through mind-centering activities such as dreaming and meditating. The third eye chakra has been perceived by spiritual traditions as being a mystical, intriguing center, which is not surprising considering it is the cosmic gateway to unlocking universal truth. It allows us to expand out of the self and the earth-based realm into an expansive dimension devoid of time.

Words associated with the third eye chakra: *concentration, dreams, illusion, imagination, indigo, insight, intuition, mood, perception, psychic ability, sleep, spiral, thought, vision, wisdom.*

CHAKRA ANATOMY AND PHYSIOLOGY

The third eye chakra, situated slightly above the space between the eyes, oversees the eyes and brain and all of their functions, including sight, balancing neurotransmitters, and regulating hormone secretion. It is largely responsible for the expression of moods and personality.

Third eye chakra anatomy: brain, eyebrows, eyes, forehead, hormone regulation, neurotransmitters, pineal gland, pituitary gland.

HEALTHY INDICATIONS

A person who is comfortable with their intuitive self is someone who follows their dreams, processes thoughts within a larger context of experience, separates truth from illusion, understands the value of heeding intuition, aligns with Divine guidance, practices loving detachment, and balances their moods.

UNHEALTHY INDICATIONS

If you answer yes to a majority of the following questions, your third eye chakra may need healing:

- *Is your dream life sometimes more real to you than your waking life?* Do you have erratic sleep patterns, like consistently sleeping less than five hours or more than nine hours, and vivid dreams, which can sometimes be disturbing and real? An imbalanced third eye chakra will reveal itself in changes in sleeping and dreaming. Those people who have haunting or extremely vivid dreams, or find themselves intrigued with other realities more than the one they live in, could have excessive activity in their third eye chakra. Reining in this activity by balancing neurotransmitters through supplementation (or through other activities like dream journaling or meditating) could help us funnel energy through this center.

- *Do you tend to be overanalytical, constantly ruminating about your decisions or reactions to situations, to the point of losing sight of the overall picture?* Do you second-guess yourself? Are you obsessive-compulsive, trying to keep your thoughts in check and your surroundings suppressed? Thoughts are within the realm of the third eye chakra. When they get the better of us, such as in the form of "monkey mind" (obsessive, bombarding thoughts), the third eye chakra needs some cleaning out and reorganization.

- *Are you prone to becoming depressed and feeling cut off from reality?* Do you have difficulty staying in the present moment, living more comfortably in your imagination or illusory life? Those with third eye chakra disturbances tend to seek ways to "get away from it all" by indulging in food or drink, particularly chocolate, coffee, or alcohol. They use drugs or have used them in the past. An addictive nature represents the involvement of third eye chakra energy.

SUPPLEMENTS FOR THE THIRD EYE CHAKRA

MACRONUTRIENTS AND MACRONUTRIENT SUPPLEMENTS

Amino Acids

Neurotransmitters are either amino acids (like glutamic acid and glycine) or made from amino acids (for example, serotonin is made from tryptophan, and dopamine, epinephrine, and norepinephrine are all synthesized from tyrosine). The amino acid methionine combines with ATP to make S-adenosylmethionine (SAM), a compound used to facilitate neurotransmitter production. As a result, it is important to incorporate healthy, complete protein sources into the diet for the broad array of essential amino acids that they provide. Animal protein, like whey protein, provides this spectrum of amino acids. These amino acids or neurotransmitter precursors help to balance the third eye chakra through their excitatory and inhibitory effects on the brain.

Essential fatty acids: Long-chain essential fats, particularly those from the omega-3 family, are needed for the third eye chakra tissues, the brain and eyes. Specifically, two fatty acids from fish, eicosapentaenoic acid (EPA, twenty carbons long) and docosahexaenoic acid (DHA, twenty-two carbons long), are most important. Taking 1 gram of EPA twice daily may improve depression, uplift mood, and provide positive changes in personality, such as reduced aggression. For schizophrenia, 1 to 3 grams (in divided doses) of EPA or of ethyl-EPA (a particular form of EPA) may be helpful in addition to existing treatment. A dose of 1 gram EPA as ethyl-EPA has been recommended for treatment of borderline personality disorder.

The other essential long-chain omega-3, DHA, is found in high concentrations in brain matter (about one-third of the brain is DHA). Infants fed breast milk containing higher levels of essential fats tend to have better cognitive outcomes in the long term than infants fed formula. DHA may reduce the risk of age-related macular degeneration, improve attention deficit hyperactivity disorder (ADHD), and improve night vision. For infant brain development, it has been recommended that pregnant women take 200 milligrams DHA daily. For improving night vision, 480 milligrams DHA has been used.

Both EPA and DHA should be taken with meals. They may interfere with the activity of anticoagulant drugs and promote internal bleeding; therefore, do not use them before, during, or after surgery.

VITAMINS

Vitamin A

See the root chakra chapter for specific details. Vitamin A is required for healthy vision. In vitamin A deficiency, night blindness can occur and, if left untreated, eventually progress to complete loss of vision. Vitamin A supplements are often taken for improving vision and for eye diseases like age-related macular degeneration, glaucoma, and cataracts.

Vitamin B1

See the solar plexus chakra chapter for specific details. Vitamin B1 helps to produce acetylcholine, an essential neurotransmitter in the brain involved in memory. Individuals with Alzheimer's disease commonly have low amounts of acetylcholine in the brain.

Vitamin B6

See the solar plexus chakra chapter for specific details. This vitamin serves as co-factor for enzymes that convert L-tryptophan to serotonin, and L-tyrosine to norepinephrine. Thus, deficiency may result in depressive symptoms or mood changes. Compared to healthy control subjects, depressed people have low vitamin B6. Vitamin B6 may play a role in psychiatric disorders and related conditions such as Alzheimer's disease, hyperactivity, learning disabilities, and anxiety. Doses of up to 100 milligrams daily may be helpful in treating premenstrual depression.

Vitamin B12

See the root chakra chapter for specific details. Vitamin B12 is used for memory loss, sleep disorders, Alzheimer's disease, depression, and psychiatric disorders. Deficiency can lead to cognitive impairment and personality and mood disorders. Daily oral doses of 2 to 5 milligrams B12 may be needed to treat deficiency, especially those who are not able to absorb this vitamin from food or who do not eat vitamin B12-rich foods (such as vegetarians). Hydrochloric acid production in the stomach is needed for vitamin B12 absorption. Since acid production decreases with age, older adults may need vitamin B12 supplementation.

Folate (Folic Acid)

See the root chakra chapter for specific details. Folate-deficiency symptoms that pertain to the brain (and third eye chakra) include depression, insomnia, forgetfulness, irritability, and anxiety. People with depression have lower blood-folate levels than control subjects, although it is unclear whether these low levels are a cause or consequence of depression. There also seems to be a relationship between high homocysteine levels and depression. Doses of 800 micrograms daily, in addition to folate from the diet, have been shown to substantially reduce levels of homocysteine in the blood.

Vitamin C

See the root chakra chapter for specific details. This water-soluble vitamin plays a crucial role in the metabolism of tyrosine (which converts to dopamine), and is a cofactor in the synthesis of norepinephrine, dopamine, and tryptophan. Psychiatric symptoms related to depression, mania, and paranoia have been shown to improve in patients taking 1 gram of ascorbic acid. Individuals with schizophrenia have benefited from vitamin C supplements, taken alone or together with omega-3 fatty acids and vitamin E.

Vitamin D

See the crown chakra chapter for specific details. Depressive symptoms and impaired cognitive ability, particularly in the elderly, have been shown to be associated with low vitamin D levels. High doses of vitamin D ameliorate depressive symptoms in depressed overweight and obese individuals.

MINERALS

Magnesium

See the heart chakra chapter for specific details. Magnesium deficiency can cause poor attention, memory loss, restlessness, insomnia, tics, and dizziness. Low levels of magnesium have been reported in depressed individuals. Subsequent magnesium supplementation improves depression. Animal studies have shown that magnesium can act as an antidepressant and antianxiety agent. It is also used to treat premenstrual mood changes and sleep disturbances associated with aging. A typical dose is 125 to 300 milligrams daily, taken with meals and at bedtime to help with depression. Magnesium, at 600 milligrams daily, has also been used to prevent migraine headaches.

BOTANICALS/OTHER

Neurotransmitter Support

Energy transmission within the realm of the third eye chakra occurs primarily through the neurotransmitter messengers, which travel from synapse to synapse, forming a bridge of communication to the crown chakra. Each of the neurotransmitters has its role, ranging from excitatory to calming, and they modulate the energy flow that controls mood, thought, memory, and cognition. In some cases, we may not have enough of the raw material (certain amino acids) used to make neurotransmitters. Other imbalances can involve inadequate vitamins or minerals, like vitamin C, to convert an amino acid to a neurotransmitter. When neurotransmitters are balanced, the third eye chakra can receive the insight it needs.

Acetyl-L-carnitine: Acetyl-L-carnitine, derived from animal foods like meat and dairy products, is structurally related to the neurotransmitter acetylcholine. It contributes chemical groups to the formation of acetylcholine and promotes its release. Supplementation of acetyl-L-carnitine may be useful in Alzheimer's disease (2 to 3 grams divided into two to three doses daily). It is well tolerated, but gastrointestinal upset and agitation may be experienced by some individuals. Interacts with anticoagulant drugs.

Choline: As discussed in the solar plexus chapter, choline is a precursor for the neurotransmitter acetylcholine. It is also found as part of the cell-membrane phospholipid (found within the brain matter), phosphatidylcholine.

5-Hydroxytryptophan (5-HTP): 5-HTP is made in the body from the amino acid L-tryptophan and is subsequently converted to serotonin. Supplementation with 5-HTP can lead to increased synthesis of serotonin, which is the reason it is used for sleep disorders, depression, anxiety, and headaches. Its safety is controversial, as there remains a concern as to whether it can cause eosinophilia myalgia syndrome (a flu-like, neurological condition that is incurable; symptoms include intense muscle pain, rashes, and breathing difficulties), when contaminants are present. Side effects may include gastrointestinal complaints. Do not combine with drugs that alter levels of serotonin. Please use under the supervision of a qualified healthcare professional. Doses of 150 to 300 milligrams daily have been used for depression.

Inositol: Like choline, inositol is incorporated into a phospholipid structure (specifically, phosphatidylinositol) that is found within all cells in the body, but particularly in the brain. Supplementation with myo-inositol (a common form of inositol synthesized in the human body) has been used for a variety of conditions. It is important to the third eye chakra because of its role in the functioning of neurotransmitter receptors and its ability to help regulate neurotransmitter release. Furthermore, it may improve obsessive-compulsive disorder, panic disorder, and depression. Although generally well tolerated, it may cause nausea, fatigue, headaches, and dizziness in some individuals. Certain drugs, such as lithium, carbamazepine, and valproic acid, can cause low levels of inositol in the brain. Doses for different third eye chakra conditions include 12 grams daily for depression, 12 to 18 grams daily for panic disorder, and 6 grams daily for lithium-induced psoriasis. *See the sacral chakra chapter for inositol's effects on fertility and the crown chakra chapter for its effects on the nervous system.*

St. John's wort *(Hypericum perforatum):* This plant, typically the flower portion, is used for its antidepressant activity, specifically its ability to influence neurotransmitter levels. Exercise caution if using it in conjunction with medications, as it induces several enzymes that metabolize drugs. Consult a healthcare professional to see whether you can take this botanical with other medications. Side effects mirror those of an overactive third eye chakra and include insomnia, vivid dreams, restlessness, irritability, dizziness, and headache, along with sensitivity to light and gastrointestinal upset. If taken with other supplements that influence neurotransmitter activity, this botanical may produce an additive effect. St. John's wort standardized to 0.3 percent hypericin has been used at a dose of 300 milligrams three times daily for mild to moderate depression. This plant helps to balance an inactive third eye chakra.

Sleep Support

Sleep provides an opportunity for the third eye chakra to recharge its energy, allowing it to process visual stimuli, thoughts, situations, and events from a day or a lifetime. Without good quality and quantity of sleep, the third eye chakra energy becomes depleted, and we are left unable to focus, concentrate, think clearly, or even regulate our mood. Specific supplements can assist the third eye chakra in making its sleep sojourn. Dreams are a window into the dimensions of the third eye chakra. As part of healing this chakra, log your dreams in a journal and reflect on their potential symbolism and meaning.

Hops *(Humulus lupulus):* Hop cones contain a volatile oil that may have sedative properties. Traditionally, the hop plant has been used to treat anxiety, insomnia, and sleep disorders, often in conjunction with other therapies, since the effects of hops are relatively mild. Side effects include depression, confusion, memory changes, hallucinations, and seizures. Do not use with alcohol or with supplements or drugs that have sedative properties. Those who have hormone-sensitive cancers are advised not to use hops, since they have estrogenic properties.

Lemon balm *(Melissa officinalis):* The leaf and leaf oil of lemon balm have calming, sedative effects. Oral extracts (and oils in aromatherapy) are used for treating anxiety, insomnia, restlessness, agitation in Alzheimer's disease, and ADHD. Side effects include gastrointestinal complaints, dizziness, and wheezing. Additive effects may occur when lemon balm is taken with other supplements or drugs that have sedative or depressant effects.

Melatonin: Melatonin is a hormone made and secreted by the pineal gland. It plays a role in sleep patterns and circadian rhythm. Its secretion is regulated by light-dark cycles. Melatonin can be taken as a dietary supplement for insomnia, jet lag, circadian rhythm disorders, Alzheimer's disease, depression, sleep-wake cycle disturbances, and cluster headaches. It is generally well tolerated, but can result in daytime drowsiness, headaches, dizziness, and even seizures in some people. Do not operate machinery for four to five hours after taking melatonin. Taking melatonin with anticoagulant and sedative drugs may intensify their effects. Avoid melatonin from animal sources (for example, animal-sourced pineal gland material) because it may contain contaminants. Doses of 0.3 to 3 milligrams at bedtime have been used for insomnia, and doses up to 9 milligrams have been used for Alzheimer's patients experiencing sleep disturbances.

Passionflower *(Passiflora incarnata):* This herb has been used for insomnia and anxiety. Side effects include dizziness, confusion, sedation, and ataxia (uncoordinated muscle movements). This botanical may interact with supplements and drugs that have sedative properties.

Valerian root *(Valeriana officinalis):* The root and rhizome of this plant has sedative, hypnotic, antianxiety, and antidepressive effects. It has been used traditionally for insomnia, reducing the time it takes to fall asleep and improving sleep quality. It has also been used to treat for anxiety, restlessness, depression, and ADHD. Valerian is often combined with other sedative herbs, like hops. Side effects include headache, excitability, insomnia, cardiac disturbance, gastric complaints, vivid dreams, and morning drowsiness. There are also reports that it causes liver toxicity. The long-term effects of valerian on liver function remain unknown; therefore, valerian is recommended for short-term use only. Exercise caution if combining valerian with other herbs or drugs that have sedative effects. Do not use with alcohol, Xanax, benzodiazepines, or central nervous system depressants. Since it may influence the metabolism of a number of drugs, use it under the supervision of a qualified health care professional. A does of 600 milligrams valerian extract has been shown to produce favorable outcomes when insomniacs took it thirty minutes before bedtime for twenty-eight days.

Eye Support

The third eye chakra is responsible for vision—not just the ability to see the outside world (via our two eyes), but also inner vision and perception of what is illusion versus truth and wisdom (the third eye, which sits slightly above and between the two eyeballs). Nutrients like vitamin A and potent-colored pigments like lutein, zeaxanthin, and bilberry are able to provide the eyes and third eye chakra with the vibration they need to see clearly. If you are experiencing visual problems, ask yourself the obvious questions: What am I not willing to see? What is clouding my vision?

Bilberry fruit extract *(Vaccinium myrtillus):* In addition to its effects on blood circulation (see the heart chakra chapter) and on blood sugar, the high concentration of purple pigments (anthocyanidins) contained within bilberry fruit may be useful for improving visual acuity and treating eye afflictions such as night vision, cataracts, and retinal conditions (particularly those related to diabetes). Please work with a qualified health care provider if you are diabetic and wish to supplement with bilberry.

Lutein (and zeaxanthin): Lutein is a yellow-pigmented carotenoid found in green-yellow vegetables, like broccoli, spinach, and kale, that typically occurs together with another carotenoid, zeaxanthin. Both lutein and zeaxanthin are highly concentrated in the human macula and retina. It is thought that they function as antioxidants, protecting the fragile eye tissue from light damage. In population studies, people with a high dietary intake of lutein have a decreased risk for developing severe cataracts and age-related macular degeneration (AMD). Studies have shown that people with AMD, cataracts, and retinal disorders benefit from lutein supplements (10 to 30 milligrams per day).

Cognition Support

The third eye chakra supports cognition by piecing together all input and synthesizing it into thought. Our ability to focus, learn, and retain information is determined by the workings of the brain and third eye chakra. If the mind is clear and uncluttered, we can concentrate more effectively. In addition to EPA and DHA, some other botanicals and nutrients can help keep the mind sharp and focused. Meditation may also be helpful for this purpose. Strengthen the mind through affirmations, mantras, and by keeping it elastic through a variety of mental activity.

Brahmi *(Bacopa monnieri):*An Ayurvedic herb commonly used to enhance learning, anxiety, memory, and reduce the symptoms of ADHD. The leaf, which contains the actives, bacosides A and B, may modulate the realease of acetylcholine (a neurotransmitter important in memory). A dose of 300 milligrams brahmi extract improved verbal learning, memory, and information processing in healthy people.

Gotu kola *(Centella asiatica):* Gotu kola has been used in traditional medicine for reducing anxiety and depression, and increasing memory and intelligence. It may work by influencing GABA (gamma-aminobutyric acid) receptors in the brain. As discussed in the heart chakra chapter, it improves blood circulation and, by doing so, stimulates brain function. Side effects may include gastrointestinal complaints, nausea, drowsiness, and liver toxicity (elevated liver enzymes). Do not use with herbs, supplements, or drugs that affect the liver or that have sedative properties. A recent study showed that 750 milligrams of a gotu kola plant extract for two months positively affected mood and cognition in an elderly population.

Phosphatidylserine: One of the most abundant phospholipids (a type of fat) in the brain, phosphatidylserine has been used for Alzheimer's disease, dementia, mental function decline, ADHD, and depression. Studies have shown that it improves attention, verbal fluency, and memory in people with age-associated cognitive decline, and improves cognition and behavior in people with Alzheimer's disease. Side effects include gastrointestinal complaints and insomnia. Avoid animal-derived sources of phosphatidylserine due to the risk for contamination. Vegetable forms, like soy-sourced phosphatidylserine, are recommended. Phosphatidylserine supplements may interact with all drugs that modify acetylcholine levels or the action of acetylcholine in the brain. The typical dose is 100 milligrams three times daily for Alzheimer's disease, dementia, or memory impairment in aging adults.

L-theanine: Theanine, an amino acid found in low levels (1 to 3 percent) in green tea, has been shown to impact brain function. Studies using human electroencephalographs (EEG, or a device used to measure the electrical activity of the brain) have shown that as little as 50 milligrams of L-theanine can promote the frequency of the alpha waves (waves that relax the mind without drowsiness) in the brain. L-theanine supplementation has been used for anxiety, Alzheimer's disease, and cognition improvement. Use with caution if taking it together with supplements or drugs that lower blood pressure, as it is thought that L-theanine can enhance this effect. For improving cognition (specifically, the ability to sustain attention to a mental task), 250 milligrams daily has been found to have favorable effects. Studies have demonstrated that when L-theanine (100 milligrams) is combined with caffeine (50 milligrams), there is significant improvement of speed and accuracy of cognitive tasks.

CHAPTER 10

SUPPLEMENTS FOR PURIFICATION AND CLARIFICATION (CROWN CHAKRA)

The Spirit of God, I realized, is exhaustless Bliss;
His body is countless tissues of light.
PARAMAHANSA YOGANANDA, *Autobiography of a Yogi*

CHAKRA DESCRIPTION

Of all the chakras, the crown chakra has the finest, most pure vibration, a vibration that provides access to our spiritual self, or the soul. It is a direct conduit to the Divine, a passage to universal consciousness, and allows us to zoom out of our everyday world into the awareness of the amazing, enormous web of life we are enmeshed in. With the crown chakra, we can comprehend and embrace the microcosm of life and the macrocosm of existence. Through this vibration, we accept the perfection of every moment, even though with earth eyes it may appear imperfect. Prayer or meditation opens this center wide to receive the flow of God. Grace can pour forth through this center, trickling through to every cell, creating interconnections among the physical and nonphysical aspects of a human being. When we take time to release ourselves from the machinations of the physical world and look at the whole cosmos by reflecting, being still, meditating or praying, we bathe our crown chakra in the awe, wonder, and magnificence of God.

Words associated with the crown chakra: *bliss, Divine consciousness, God, highest self, infinite, interconnectedness, purity, purpose, radiance, soul, source, spirit, spirituality, unity, universe, universal truth.*

CHAKRA ANATOMY AND PHYSIOLOGY

The crown chakra, composed of fine energy, is the unifier of the entire being, linking its existence and its purpose, its function and its intelligence. This chakra's energy animates the cells by providing life-force and electrical energy through the central nervous system, allowing the organism to make its way in the world as a Divine creature.

Crown chakra anatomy: cellular intelligence, central nervous system, life force (chi, prana).

HEALTHY INDICATIONS

A person who is comfortable with their spiritual, unified self is someone who trusts their highest self; believes confidently in a higher power; surrenders their life to their soul's mission; integrates their earthly being and their spirit self; connects to spiritual beings such as angels, spirit guides, and avatars; is in tune with universal consciousness; and devotes their life to a greater purpose. An image of someone who has attained these degrees of development might fall in the category of a saint or guru, but may also be someone who goes relatively unnoticed by serving people in subtle, selfless ways like making their life's mission feeding the poor or taking care of the sick. We can develop this vibration and call to a higher purpose by finding some aspect of our lives that feeds the soul aspect of who we are: that may vary person to person and become fleshed out in song, food, words, that are used to serve others, to name a few.

UNHEALTHY INDICATIONS

If you answer yes to a majority of the following questions, your crown chakra may need healing:

- *Are you overly preoccupied with your nonearthly self?* Do you tend to live by such devout religious or spiritual tenets that you neglect your physical body to the extent you have difficulty surviving? Do you neglect your physical body by not taking care of it (such as forgetting to eat or refusing to exercise)? An overactive crown chakra may result in a priorities shift that may not benefit the entire self. When we don't treat the body as a temple or a Divine vehicle, we neglect part of us that is essential for living on this planet. Or, on the other hand, do you feel isolated or without an intimate connection to a force or being that is greater than yourself? Do you feel deep despair over the purpose of living, or feel that God has let you down, so to speak? Shutting down the crown chakra may result in a life that feels devoid of purpose due to the lack of interconnection with all of physical and spiritual life.

- *Do you find yourself struggling to make your religious or spiritual beliefs known to others?* Crown chakra issues may involve not being willing to accept that others have different beliefs than you, or openly or secretly resenting that they do. Rather than being energetically pliable and open to a connection with God, the crown chakra can take on an air of righteousness or the belief that there is a "correct" way to believe in something greater.

- *Do you find yourself constantly questioning your existence, or deny seeing yourself as more than just your physical body?* On the other end of the spectrum, denying that there is a greater spiritual force that animates us could also reflect stagnant crown chakra energy. People may avoid a spiritual path because it may alter their life, and they fear they could not accept the changes.

SUPPLEMENTS FOR THE CROWN CHAKRA

MACRONUTRIENTS AND MACRONUTRIENT SUPPLEMENTS

Purification is a pivotal crown chakra element. Whatever can help the body remove toxins resonates with the crown chakra and helps it facilitate a more seamless fit between body and spirit. This process may involve the assistance of other body tissues, like the skin (root chakra); the extracellular matrix, kidneys, and colon (sacral chakra); the liver and small intestine (solar plexus); and the lungs (heart chakra). Detoxification programs that focus on using various modalities, including dietary supplements, may keep the body collective harmonized and the crown chakra resonating at its high vibration. Examples of supplements include (1) insoluble and soluble fibers for trapping toxins in the gut and carrying them out of the body (see the sacral chakra chapter), (2) liver support to optimize the internal transformation of toxic substances and their eventual excretion (see the solar plexus chakra chapter), (3) alkalizing minerals like magnesium and potassium to assist the kidneys in efficiently releasing toxins in the urine.

Hypoallergenic powders for detoxification: Powdered supplements that are hypoallergenic (devoid of the top eight allergens: milk, eggs, peanuts, tree nuts, fish, shellfish, soy, and wheat; often made from rice since it is hypoallergenic) and expressly address the detoxification of the body by cleansing the liver or the gut would be helpful for this chakra and ultimately beneficial for the all of the chakras.

Essential fatty acids

The central nervous system is rich in the essential omega-6 and omega-3 fats. As noted in the sacral and third eye chakra chapters, these important fats are integrated throughout the body and are needed for the body to function normally. With respect to the crown chakra, adequate intake of these fats is needed for the development of nerve cells in the fetus.

Omega-6 fatty acids: The omega-6 fat, gamma-linolenic acid (GLA), is important for nerve membrane structure. It is conceivable that deficiency or reduced levels could lead to neuropathy. The human studies investigating GLA supplementation for diabetic neuropathy showed that 360 to 480 milligrams GLA for six months to one year resulted in better nerve-function scores. Animal studies with diabetic rats showed that GLA improved nerve health and nerve blood flow.

Omega-3 fatty acids: Like omega-6 fats, omega-3 fats, particularly the long-chain fats from fish and algae, EPA and DHA (see the sacral and third eye chakra chapters for more specifics), are important for nerve-cell membrane composition and for healthy blood flow to nerve cells. Diabetics with nerve pain who supplemented with 1,800 milligrams EPA for forty-eight weeks experienced reduced coldness and numbness and better nerve symptoms. Compared with olive oil, fish oil (comprised of both EPA and DHA) led to nerve regeneration in diabetic rats. Combined EPA-DHA supplementation holds promise for those with chronic nerve-degeneration conditions and may also be of benefit in acute nerve injuries.

VITAMINS

Multivitamin

Multivitamins contain a broad spectrum of nutritional substances for the entire body. Therefore, they are excellent for balancing and integrating the whole being. Of course, they are not meant to take the place of a balanced diet. They are meant to supply the body with small amounts of nutrients that will subtly supplement any shortcomings based on day-to-day dietary variation. With the added stress of the polluted, toxic environment we live in, it is essential that we have added "vibrational insurance." Since a multivitamin is often taken on a daily basis, it should ideally be free of unessential preservatives, fats, dyes, and sweeteners, such as the following: sucralose (Splenda®), any of the FD&C (Food, Drug, and Cosmetic) colors, hydrogenated oils, and BHT (butylated hydroxytoluene). If you have an allergy to corn, avoid multivitamins that contain cornstarch or maltodextrin (often corn derived).

Biotin

See the root chakra chapter for more specific details. Biotin deficiency (relatively rare, but can occur with malabsorption syndromes, pregnancy, long-term parenteral nutrition, and diabetes) can lead to neurological symptoms such as tingling or prickling sensations or numbness (a condition referred to as paresthesia). Lower than normal levels of biotin have been found in the cerebrospinal fluid (fluid in the spinal column) and blood of people with multiple sclerosis and epilepsy compared to people without these conditions. In a small study with people on dialysis (a procedure that removes toxins from blood, commonly done for kidney failure or other kidney issues) that had peripheral neuropathy, 10 milligrams of biotin, taken in divided doses throughout the day for one to four years, resulted in improved paresthesia, restless legs, and ability to walk.

Vitamin B1 (thiamin, benfotiamine)

See the solar plexus chapter for specific details. Thiamin deficiency typically results in neurological symptoms. Chronic alcohol use (which energetically causes shifts in our reality and a lack of cohesion between body and spirit) can result in thiamin deficiency and, ultimately, neuropathy. The fat-soluble form of thiamin, called benfotiamine, has been touted as the preferred compound (relative to its water-soluble form) for promoting nerve-cell health in neuropathic conditions, particularly since the outer membrane of nerve cells is made of fat. Human studies have demonstrated that benfotiamine may be helpful in relieving pain in individuals with peripheral neuropathy when taken at 400 milligrams daily (two 50 milligrams tablets taken four times throughout the day). Benfotiamine may work synergistically with a B-vitamin complex.

Vitamin B6

See the solar plexus chapter for specific details. This essential B vitamin has a unique relationship with neuropathies: its deficiency is associated with the development of peripheral neuropathy (neuropathy in the extremities), while high doses (1 to 5 grams daily) may cause peripheral neuropathy. Therefore, it has the ability to support a deficient crown chakra, but can also lead to excessive energy in this energetic region.

Vitamin B12

See the root chakra chapter for specific details. Vitamin B12 is used as an antiaging agent and for tremors. Deficiency results in neurological damage, including impaired myelin (fatty sheath around nerves) production, and may lead to nerve-cell damage. High levels of neurotoxic inflammatory compounds (called cytokines) and decreased levels of nerve-supporting factors (growth factors) have been found with B12 deficiency. Testing levels of homocysteine in the blood may help to identify those at risk for deficiency.

Vitamin C

See the root chakra chapter for specific details. Vitamin C deficiency can result in nervous-system dysfunction. Nerve cells grow in the presence of vitamin C. When administered alone or together with vitamin E, vitamin C can prevent decreased nerve conduction that occurs under cold-temperature extremes. Both these vitamins help to reverse age-related neuron changes.

Vitamin D

See the root chakra chapter for specific details. Although the primary function of vitamin D connects most closely with the root chakra, due to its involvement with calcium and bone structure, this vitamin also extends to the realm of the crown chakra because of its nature: It can be derived through sunshine, and every cell in the body has a receptor for vitamin D. It also acts like a hormone throughout the body, creating alignment within body systems. It may play a role in preventing nerve degeneration and in conditions that involve the nervous and immune systems (such as multiple sclerosis).

Vitamin E

See the sacral chakra chapter for specific details. Vitamin E deficiency (associated with intestinal diseases and malabsorption) may lead to neurological symptoms. When people with diabetic neuropathy were given 900 milligrams of vitamin E for six months, their nerve function improved more than the group not given vitamin E. It may also help with the neurotoxicity caused by chemotherapy.

MINERALS

Magnesium

Diabetics typically have lower magnesium than healthy people. A daily dose of 300 milligrams given to magnesium-deficient type 1 diabetics was able to prevent the progressive worsening of neuropathic symptoms.

Nervous System Support

The crown chakra's energy permeates the entire human body landscape through the intricate web of the nervous system. If nerves are damaged or degenerating (neuropathic), they might cause pain, numbness, and tingling sensations—all of which can be debilitating. From a physiological aspect, these effects can occur because of chronic diseases like diabetes, exposure to environmental toxins, alcoholism, or nutritional deficiencies, or they can be side effects of a medication. From a spiritual (crown chakra) perspective, nerve issues may symbolize how we approach our personal divinity and how we accept spirituality in our lives. Perhaps the nerve pain is a blaring signal to pay attention to interconnectedness and communication between the body and soul. Numbness may represent a withholding or cutting ourselves off from our spiritual nature, divorcing ourselves from the soul essence of our being.

Acetyl-L-carnitine: *See the third eye chakra chapter for specific details.* Through its effects on the central nervous system, acetyl-L-carnitine assists the crown chakra in a variety of ways. It can protect nerve cells from damage, promote communication between nerves (neurotransmission), and enhance energy production in nerve cells. Animal studies indicate it may help the nerve cells to function better when under conditions of low oxygen (hypoxia). Acetyl-L-carnitine supplements can be particularly beneficial when coupled with alpha-lipoic acid. Individuals with multiple sclerosis who were given acetyl-L-carnitine had lower levels of reactive, damaging compounds in their cerebrospinal fluid compared with MS patients that did not take the supplements or people with neurological conditions not involving inflammation. Side effects include nausea, vomiting, gastrointestinal complaints, restlessness, and fishy-smelling urine, breath, and sweat. Do not take acetyl-L-carnitine together with anticoagulants, or use if you are hypothyroid or susceptible to seizures. For diabetic neuropathy, 1,500 to 3,000 milligrams daily in divided doses has been used therapeutically.

Alpha-lipoic acid: *See the solar plexus chakra chapter for specific details.* Perhaps due to its role as a lipid antioxidant (protecting fats in the body from damage by oxygen by acting as a free radical scavenger), alpha-lipoic acid, commonly found in meats and a variety of vegetables, has been shown to protect nerves from inflammation and toxicity. Oral intake has been helpful for neuropathy in the legs and feet. Side effects may include nausea and skin rash. Avoid using it with supplements and drugs that lower blood sugar. Alpha-lipoic acid may decrease the effectiveness of chemotherapy. Doses of 600 to 1,800 milligrams daily may alleviate symptoms of diabetic neuropathy, such as burning, pain, numbness, and prickling in the feet and legs.

Choline: *See the solar plexus chakra chapter for specific details.* Choline is highly concentrated in nerve tissue. Supplementation with choline during pregnancy may positively affect the developing fetus by having an impact on the structure of neurons that play a role in memory. Additionally, choline may help prevent neural-tube defects.

Coenzyme Q10: *See the heart chakra chapter for specific details.* This potent antioxidant may protect against nerve damage produced by lack of oxygen, accumulation of plaque in the arteries, and injury. Studies with people that have early stage Parkinson's disease show that they may benefit with supplementation of 300 to 1,200 milligrams daily.

Gotu kola *(Centella asiatica)*: In the Ayurvedic tradition, gotu kola has a reputation as a spiritual herb. In addition to its effects on the mind and on blood circulation, it may also affect longevity and the healing of nerve cells, as it has been shown to accelerate the repair of damaged nerve cells. Side effects may include gastrointestinal complaints, nausea, drowsiness, and liver toxicity (elevated liver enzymes). Do not use with herbs, supplements, or drugs that affect the liver or that have sedative properties. *See heart and third eye chakra chapters for its other uses.*

Inositol: Inositol is situated within specific lipids (phospholipids) of nerve-cell membranes. Low levels of myo-inositol (the form of inositol in the human body) in nerve cells have been associated with the underlying dysfunction related to diabetic neuropathy. In animal studies, ingested myo-inositol prevented nerve degeneration. In a small human study, nerve myo-inositol levels were found to be lower in people with diabetic neuropathy compared to those without the condition. Finally, in people with normal or abnormal blood-sugar balance, high levels of nerve myo-inositol were connected with better nerve cell health (indicated by increased nerve fiber density). *See the sacral chakra chapter for inositol's effects on fertility and the third eye chakra chapter for its effects on the brain.*

Aging Support

Achieving vitality, as measured by life quality and length, is one of the hallmarks of the crown chakra. Aiming for mastery of the mind and body has been part of the daily practice of ancient gurus. The ability to control bodily functions, and ultimately our aging process, indicates that the crown chakra is in full, lotuslike bloom. Of course, a variety of practices—such as deep breathing (a full acceptance and merging with all of life), yoga (integrating body and mind), and eating pure, clean foods, as well as including supplements that enhance the overall energy vibration of the body (and spirit)—can help.

Resveratrol: Resveratrol is a natural compound found in the skin and leaves of grapes. Cell and animal studies demonstrate that many of the health-promoting qualities of red wine, such as its ability to reduce inflammation, reduce platelet aggregation, serve as an antioxidant and anticancer compound, and favorably modify fat metabolism, stem from the resveratrol found in the wine. Specific to the crown chakra, resveratrol appears to protect nerve cells from damage and death from inflammation, as shown in cell and animal studies. Newer research involving various organisms (from yeast to rodents) suggests that it can activate enzymes in the body (sirtuins) that mimic the effects of caloric restriction; the outcome has been decreased aging and onset of age-related diseases, as well as lifespan extension. Research is still lacking regarding resveratrol's effects in humans and its ability to prolong human lifespan. If you are taking resveratrol, note that it acts as a phytoestrogen (see the chapter on the sacral chakra) and may intensify estrogen's effects in the body. Therefore, individuals with hormone-sensitive conditions, such as breast, uterine, ovarian cancer, as well as endometriosis and fibroids, should avoid or use this supplement under the guidance of a qualified healthcare professional. Do not take it together with supplements or drugs that have anticoagulant properties. Additionally, resveratrol can influence how the body metabolizes certain drugs.

APPENDIX A

Chakras and Corresponding Herbs and Supplements

Chakras	Root	Sacral	Solar Plexus	Heart	Throat	Third Eye	Crown
VITAMINS							
B-Complex			☼				
Biotin	✻		☼				✻
Folic acid	☼	✻		✻		✻	
Multivitamin	✻	✻	✻	✻	✻	✻	☼
Vitamin A	☼	✻	✻	✻	✻	✻	
Vitamin B1 (thiamin, water soluble)			☼			✻	✻
Vitamin B1 (benfotiamine, fat soluble)							☼
Vitamin B12 (cyanocobalamin)	☼		✻	✻		✻	✻
Vitamin B2 (riboflavin)	✻		☼				
Vitamin B3 (niacin)			☼	✻			
Vitamin B5 (pantothenic acid)	✻		☼				
Vitamin B6 (pyridoxine)	✻	✻	☼	✻		✻	✻
Vitamin C (ascorbic acid)	☼				✻	✻	✻
Vitamin D (cholecalciferol)	☼				✻	✻	✻
Vitamin E (tocopherols)		☼		✻		✻	✻
Vitamin K (phylloquinone)	✻		☼				
MINERALS							
Calcium	☼	✻		✻		✻	✻
Chromium			☼				
Copper	☼						

Chakras	Root	Sacral	Solar Plexus	Heart	Throat	Third Eye	Crown
Iodine				●	☆		
Iron	☆						
Magnesium	●	●	●	☆	●	●	●
Phosphorus	☆	●	●			●	
Potassium				☆		●	●
Selenium	●	☆				●	
Zinc	☆					●	
OTHER							
5-hydroxytryptophan (5-HTP)						☆	
Acetyl-L-carnitine						☆	
Aloe vera		☆					
Alpha-lipoic acid			☆				●
Amino acids (protein)	☆					●	
Andrographis	☆				●		
Ashwagandha	☆		●				
Astragalus	☆				●		
Bacopa monnieri						☆	
Bearberry		☆					
Beta-carotene	●	☆					
Betaine hydrochloride	●		☆				
Bilberry fruit extract				☆		●	
Bioflavonoids				☆			
Bitter melon			☆				
Black cohosh		☆					
Blue-green algae					☆		
Bromelain	●		☆		●		
Butterbur					☆		
Cat's claw	☆						

Chakras	Root	Sacral	Solar Plexus	Heart	Throat	Third Eye	Crown
Chasteberry fruit		☼					
Choline			☼			✸	✸
Chondroitin sulfate	☼						
Cinnamon			☼				
Coenzyme Q10				☼			✸
Cordyceps	☼		✸				
Cranberry extract		☼					
Dandelion root			☼				
Dang shen	☼		✸				
Digestive enzymes	✸	✸	☼				
Docosahexaenoic acid (DHA)		☼		✸		✸	✸
Echinacea	☼				✸		
Eicosapentaenoic acid (EPA)	✸	☼		✸		✸	✸
Elderberry	☼				✸		
Eleutherococcus senticosus	☼		✸				
Fenugreek			☼				
Fish oils		☼		✸		✸	✸
Garlic				☼			
Ginger root	✸		☼				
Ginseng, American	✸		☼				
Ginseng, Panax	☼		✸				
Glucosamine sulfate	☼				✸		
Gotu kola				☼		✸	✸
Grape seed extract				☼			
Green food powders				☼			
Green tea extract		☼				✸	
Gymnema			☼				

Chakra	Root	Sacral	Solar Plexus	Heart	Throat	Third Eye	Crown
Hawthorn				☆			
Hesperidin				☆			
Holy basil	☆		✸				
Hops	✸					☆	
Horse chestnut				☆			
Indian frankincense	☆						
Indole-3-carbinol/DIM				☆			
Inositol (myo-inositol)		✸				☆	✸
L-arginine	☆			✸			
L-carnitine	✸	✸	☆				
Lemon balm						☆	
L-theanine						☆	
Licorice	☆		✸		✸		
Lutein						☆	
Lycopene	☆			✸			
Marshmallow					☆		
Melatonin						☆	
Methylsulfonylmethane (MSM)	☆				✸		
Milk thistle			☆				
Passionflower						☆	
Phosphatidylserine						☆	
Phytosterols	✸			☆			
Plant oils		☆				✸	✸
Prebiotics	✸	☆	✸				
Probiotics	✸	☆			✸		
Quercetin				☆			

Chakras	Root	Sacral	Solar Plexus	Heart	Throat	Third Eye	Crown
Red clover		☆					
Red yeast rice				☆			
Reishi	☆		★				
Resveratrol							☆
Rhodiola	☆		★				
Rutin				☆			
Saw palmetto	☆						
Schisandra	☆		★				
Sea kelp					☆		
Slippery elm					☆		
Soy isoflavones		☆		★			
Soy protein	☆			★			
St. John's wort						☆	
Stinging nettle					☆		
Turmeric	★		☆				
Valerian root						☆	
Willow bark	☆						
Zeaxanthin						☆	

APPENDIX B

Chakra Reference Guide to Physiological Conditions

☼: primary chakra affected; ✹: secondary chakra(s) affected

Chakras	Root	Sacral	Solar Plexus	Heart	Throat	Third Eye	Crown
Condition							
Adrenal gland dysfunction	☼		☼			✹	
Aging/oxidative stress	✹	✹	✹				☼
Allergic rhinitis	✹				☼		
Altered taste perception					☼		
Anemia	☼			✹			
Blood-lipid abnormalities				☼			
Blood-sugar imbalance			☼				
Bone disorders	☼						
Breast health		✹		☼			
Circulation disorders	☼			☼			
Common cold	☼			✹	✹		
Depression	✹					☼	☼
Digestive tract dysfunction	✹	✹	☼				
Fatigue/low energy production	✹		☼			✹	
Hearing loss					☼	✹	
Hormonal conditions		☼		✹			
Immune disorders	☼				✹		✹

Chakras	Root	Sacral	Solar Plexus	Heart	Throat	Third Eye	Crown
Condition							
Infections	✿				✹		
Inflammatory conditions	✿	✹	✹				
Insomnia						✿	
Liver dysfunction			✿				
Low stomach acid production (achlorhydria)	✹		✿				
Memory loss						✿	✹
Nervous system disorders						✹	✿
Stomach upset			✿				
Prostate health	✿						
Protein maldigestion	✹		✿				
Sore throat	✹				✿		
Thyroid dysfunction					✿		
Urinary tract conditions	✹	✿					
Wound healing	✿						

APPENDIX C

Recommended Vitamin and Mineral Intakes for Adult Men and Women

VITAMINS	DRI[a] Men	Women	TUL[b]	Comments
Vitamin A	900 mcg (3,000 IU)	700 mcg (2,333 IU)	3,000 mcg (10,000 IU)	Daily intakes of greater than or equal to 10,000 units shown to increase risk for osteoporosis and hip fractures in postmenopausal women.
Biotin	30 mcg	30 mcg	ND	
Vitamin B1 (Thiamin)	1.2 mg	1.1 mg	ND	
Vitamin B2 (Riboflavin)	1.3 mg	1.1 mg	ND	Those under stress or who exercise frequently may need more riboflavin.
Vitamin B3 (Niacin)	16 mg	14 mg	35 mg[c]	Daily doses of 1,200–3,000 milligrams of niacin have been used to help normalize blood fats.
Pantothenic acid	5 mg	5 mg	ND	Daily doses of 100–500 millligrams have been recommended for those who experience chronic stress.
Vitamin B6 (Pyridoxine)	1.7 mg	1.5 mg	100 mg	Daily doses of 50–100 mg used for PMS.
Folic acid	400 mcg	400 mcg	1,000 mcg[c]	Daily doses higher than 1,000 micrograms not advised due to potential for masking vitamin B12 deficiency. It is recommended that women able to become pregnant consume 400 mcg folic acid from dietary supplements or fortified foods in addition to eating food sources of folate.

	DRI[a]		TUL[b]	Comments
	Men	**Women**		
Vitamin B12	2.4 mcg	2.4 mcg	ND	Vegetarians and individuals with poor digestion (particularly adults older than fifty) need to ensure that they consume foods high in vitamin B12 or take a dietary supplement.
Vitamin C	90 mg	75 mg	2,000 mg	Increased daily amounts, as much as 600–1,000 mg, have been used in preventing the common cold and for high stress conditions.
Vitamin D	15 mcg (600 IU)	15 mcg (600 IU)	50 mcg (2,000 IU)	The amount of vitamin D obtained naturally through the skin may change throughout the year with varying periods of sunlight, and, therefore, alter diet and dietary supplement requirements.
Vitamin E	15 mg	15 mg	1,000 mg[c]	
Vitamin K	120 mcg	90 mcg	ND	
Choline	550 mg	425 mg	3,500 mg	
MINERALS				
Calcium	1,300 mg	1,300 mg	2,500 mg	Daily doses of 1,000–1,600 mg elemental calcium have been used for preventing osteoporosis in postmenopausal women. Absorption can be enhanced when taken together with vitamin D.
Chromium	35 mcg	25 mcg	ND	Daily doses as high as 200–1,000 micrograms in divided doses throughout the day have been recommended for individuals with type 2 diabetes.
Copper	0.9 mg	0.9 mg	10 mg	
Iodine	150 mcg	150 mcg	1,100 mcg	In addition to its use for the thyroid gland, iodine (80 mcg per kilogram body weight of molecular iodine) has been used for fibrocystic breast disease.

	DRI[a]		TUL[b]	Comments
	Men	Women		
Iron	11 mg	18 mg	45 mg	
Magnesium	420 mg	360 mg	350 mg[d]	
Phosphorus	1,250 mg	1,250 mg[c]	4,000 mg	
Selenium	55 mcg	55 mcg	400 mcg	
Zinc	11 mg	9 mg	40 mg	

[a]Dietary Reference Intakes (DRI) were established from 1997 to 2001 by the Food and Nutrition Board of the Institute of Medicine, National Academies. Note that in some cases there is a range of DRI values over the adult lifecycle. Only the highest value is presented in this table. Values for pregnancy and lactation are not included.

[b]The tolerable upper limit (TUL) is the upper level of intake (represents total intake from food, water, and supplements) considered to be safe and likely to pose no risk of side effects. Amounts that exceed the UL may result in a greater propensity towards side effects.

ND: not determined

[c]Applies to forms obtained from dietary supplements, fortified foods, or a combination of both.

[d]Does not include magnesium from food or water.

Sources:

Table modified from the Council of Responsible Nutrition's tables, "Comparison of Current RDIs, New DRIs, and ULs for Vitamins" *(www.crnusa.org/about_recs.html)* and "Comparison of Current RDIs, New DRIs, and ULs for Minerals" *(www.crnusa.org/about_recs2.html)*.

Dietary Reference Intakes for Calcium, Phosphorous, Magnesium, Vitamin D, and Fluoride (1997)

Dietary Reference Intakes for Thiamin, Riboflavin, Niacin, Vitamin B6, Folate, Vitamin B12, Pantothenic Acid, Biotin, and Choline (1998)

Dietary Reference Intakes for Vitamin C, Vitamin E, Selenium, and Carotenoids (2000)

Dietary Reference Intakes for Vitamin A, Vitamin K, Arsenic, Boron, Chromium, Copper, Iodine, Iron, Manganese, Molybdenum, Nickel, Silicon, Vanadium, and Zinc (2001)

These reports may be accessed via *www.nap.edu.*

Institute of Medicine. Food and Nutrition Board. "Dietary Reference Intakes: Recommended Intakes for Individuals." Copyright © 2004 by the National Academy of Sciences.

Available on the United States Department of Agriculture, National Agricultural Library, Food and Nutrition Information Center website at *www.iom.edu/Object.File/Master/21/372/0.pdf.*

BIBLIOGRAPHY

GENERAL

Balch JF, Balch PA. *Prescription for Nutritional Healing.* New York: Avery Publishing Group, 1990.

Haas EM. *Staying Healthy with Nutrition.* Berkeley: Celestial Arts, 2006.

Jellin JM, ed. *Natural Medicines Comprehensive Database.* Available at: *www.naturaldatabase.com.*

Murray M, Pizzorno J. *Encyclopedia of Natural Medicine.* Rocklin: Prima Publishing, 1998.

Stargrove MB, Treasure J, McKee DL. *Herb, Nutrient, and Drug Interactions.* St. Louis, MO: Elsevier, 2008.

U.S. National Library of Medicine and National Institutes of Health. *PubMed* (online database). Available at: *www.ncbi.nlm.nih.gov/pubmed/*

The following sources are listed in the order in which they appear in the book.

Chapter 3

Council for Responsible Nutrition. "Dietary Supplements: Safe, Beneficial and Regulated." Available at: *www.crnusa.org/CRNRegQandA.html*

Chapter 4 (Root Chakra)

Feskanich D, Singh V, Willett WC, et al. Vitamin A intake and hip fractures among post-menopausal women. *JAMA.* 2002;287:47–54.

Cumming RG, Mitchell P, Smith W. Diet and cataract: the Blue Mountains Eye Study. *Ophthalmology.* 2000;10:450–6.

Melhus H, Michaelsson K, Kindmark A, et al. Excessive dietary intake of vitamin A is associated with reduced bone mineral density and increased risk for hip fracture. *Ann Intern Med.* 1998;129:770–8.

Food and Nutrition Board, Institute of Medicine. *Dietary Reference Intakes for Vitamin A, Vitamin K, Arsenic, Boron, Chromium, Copper, Iodine, Iron, Manganese, Molybdenum, Nickel, Silicon, Vanadium, and Zinc.* Washington, DC: National Academy Press, 2002. Available at: *books.nap.edu/030907279/html/.*

Food and Nutrition Board, Institute of Medicine. *Dietary Reference Intakes for Thiamin, Riboflavin, Niacin, Vitamin B6, Folate, Vitamin B12, Pantothenic Acid, Biotin, and Choline.* Washington, DC: National Academy Press, 2000. Available at: *books.nap.edu/books/0309065542/html/.*

Douglas RM, Chalker EB, Treacy B. Vitamin C for preventing and treating the common cold. *Cochrane Database Syst Rev.* 2000;2:CD000980.

Hemila H. Vitamin C and common cold incidence: a review of studies with subjects under heavy physical stress. *Int J Sports Med.* 1996;17:379–83.

Food and Nutrition Board, Institute of Medicine. *Dietary Reference Intakes for Vitamin C, Vitamin E, Selenium, and Carotenoids.* Washington, DC: National Academy Press, 2000. Available at: *books.nap.edu/0309069351/html/.*

Bischoff-Ferrari HA, Willett WC, Wong JB, et al. Fracture prevention with vitamin D supplementation: a meta-analysis of randomized controlled trials. *JAMA* 2005;293:2257–64.

Dawson-Hughes B, Heaney RP, Holick MF, et al. Estimates of optimal vitamin D status. *Osteoporos Int.* 2005;16:713–6.

Food and Nutrition Board, Institute of Medicine. *Dietary Reference Intakes for Calcium, Phosphorus, Magnesium, Vitamin D, and Fluoride.* Washington, DC: National Academy Press, 1999. Available at: *books.nap.edu/books/0309063507/html/.*

Bour NJS, Soullier BA, Zemel MB. Effect of level and form of phosphorus and level of calcium intake on zinc, iron, and copper bioavailability in man. *Nutr Res.* 1984;4:371–9.

Food and Nutrition Board, Institute of Medicine. *Dietary Reference Intakes for Vitamin A, Vitamin K, Arsenic, Boron, Chromium, Copper, Iodine, Iron, Manganese, Molybdenum, Nickel, Silicon, Vanadium, and Zinc.* Washington, DC: National Academy Press, 2002. Available at: *www.books.nap.edu/0309072794/html/.*

Strause L, Saltman P, Smith KT, et al. Spinal bone loss in postmenopausal women supplemented with calcium and trace minerals. *J Nutr.* 1994;124:1060–4.

Griffith DP, Liff DA, Ziegler TR, et al. Acquired copper deficiency: a potentially serious and preventable complication following gastric bypass surgery. *Obesity* (Silver Spring). 2009 Apr;17(4):827-31. Epub 2009 Jan 15.

Sengupta K, Alluri KV, Satish AR, et al. A double blind, randomized, placebo controlled study of the efficacy and safety of 5-Loxin for treatment of osteoarthritis of the knee. *Arthritis Res Ther.* 2008;10(4):R85. Epub 2008 Jul 30.

Piscoya J, Rodriguez Z, Bustamante SA, et al. Efficacy and safety of freeze-dried cat's claw in osteoarthritis of the knee: mechanisms of action of the species *Uncaria guianensis. Inflamm Res.* 2001;50:442–8.

Lukaczer D, Darland G, Tripp M, et al. A pilot trial evaluating Meta050, a proprietary combination of reduced iso-alpha acids, rosemary extract and oleanolic acid in patients with arthritis and fibromyalgia. *Phytother Res.* 2005 Oct;19(10):864–9.

Minich DM, Bland JS, Katke J, et al. Clinical safety and efficacy of NG440: a novel combination of rho iso-alpha acids from hops, rosemary, and oleanolic acid for inflammatory conditions. *Can J Physiol Pharmacol.* 2007 Sep;85(9):872–83.

Kimmatkar N, Thawani V, Hingorani L, et al. Efficacy and tolerability of *Boswellia serrata* extract in treatment of osteoarthritis of knee—a randomized double blind placebo controlled trial. *Phytomedicine.* 2003;10:3–7.

Sander O, Herborn G, Rau R. [Is H15 (resin extract of *Boswellia serrata*, "incense") a useful supplement to established drug therapy of chronic polyarthritis? Results of a double-blind pilot study]. [Article in German]. *Z Rheumatol.* 1998;57:11–16.

Chrubasik S, Eisenberg E, Balan E, et al. Treatment of low back pain exacerbations with willow bark extract: a randomized double-blind study. *Am J Med.* 2000;109:9-14.

Braham R, Dawson B, Goodman C. The effect of glucosamine supplementation on people experiencing regular knee pain. *Br J Sports Med.* 2003;37:45–9.

Houpt JB, McMillan R, Wein C, et al. Effect of glucosamine hydrochloride in the treatment of pain of osteoarthritis of the knee. *J Rheumatol.* 1999;26:2423–30.

Clegg DO, Reda DJ, Harris CL, et al. Glucosamine, chondroitin sulfate, and the two in combination for painful knee osteoarthritis. *N Engl J Med.* 2006;354:795–808.

Uebelhart D, Thonar EJ, Delmas PD, et al. Effects of oral chondroitin sulfate on the progression of knee osteoarthritis: a pilot study. *Osteoarthritis Cartilage.* 1998;6:39–46.

Bourgeois P, Chales G, Dehais J, et al. Efficacy and tolerability of chondroitin sulfate 1200 mg/day vs chondroitin sulfate 3 x 400 mg/day vs placebo. *Osteoarthritis Cartilage.* 1998;6:25–30.

Mazieres B, Combe B, Phan Van A, et al. Chondroitin sulfate in osteoarthritis of the knee: a prospective, double blind, placebo controlled multicenter clinical study. *J Rheumatol.* 2001;28:173–81.

Usha PR, Naidu MUR. Randomised, double-blind, parallel, placebo-controlled study of oral glucosamine, methylsulfonylmethane and their combinations. *Clin Drug Invest.* 2004;24:353–63.

Kim LS, Axelrod LJ, Howard P, et al. Efficacy of methylsulfonylmethane (MSM) in osteoarthritis pain of the knee: a pilot clinical trial. *Osteoarthritis Cartilage.* 2006;14:286–94.

Barrager E, Veltmann JR Jr, Schauss AG, et al. A multicentered, open-label trial on the safety and efficacy of methylsulfonylmethane in the treatment of seasonal allergic rhinitis. *J Altern Complement Med.* 2002;8:167–73.

Caceres DD, Hancke JL, Burgos RA, et al. Prevention of common colds with *Andrographis paniculata* dried extract: a pilot, double-blind trial. *Phytomedicine.* 1997;4:101–4.

Melchoir J, Spasov AA, Ostrovskij OV, et al. Double-blind, placebo-controlled pilot and phase III study of activity of standardized *Andrographis paniculata* Herba Nees extract fixed combination (Kan Jang) in the treatment of uncomplicated upper-respiratory tract infection. *Phytomedicine.* 2000;7:341–50.

Upton R, ed. *Astragalus Root: Analytical, Quality Control, and Therapeutic Monograph.* Santa Cruz, CA: American Herbal Pharmacopoeia, 1999.

Zakay-Rones Z, Thom E, Wollan T, et al. Randomized study of the efficacy and safety of oral elderberry extract in the treatment of influenza A and B virus infections. *J Int Med Res.* 2004;32:132–40.

Mohanty NK, Saxena S, Singh UP, et al. Lycopene as a chemopreventive agent in the treatment of high-grade prostate intraepithelial neoplasia. *Urol Oncol.* 2005;23:383–5.

Karppi J, Kurl S, Nurmi T, et al. Serum Lycopene and the Risk of Cancer: The Kuopio Ischaemic Heart Disease Risk Factor (KIHD) Study. *Ann Epidemiol.* 2009 May 12. [Epub ahead of print]

Kucuk O, Sarkar FH, Sakr W, et al. Phase II randomized clinical trial of lycopene supplementation before radical prostatectomy. *Cancer Epidemiol Biomarkers Prev.* 2001;10:861–8.

Giovannucci E, Rimm EB, Liu Y, et al. A prospective study of tomato products, lycopene, and prostate cancer risk. *J Natl Cancer Inst.* 2002;94:391–8.

Forbes K, Gillette K, Sehgal I. Lycopene increases urokinase receptor and fails to inhibit growth or connexin expression in a metastatically passaged prostate cancer cell line: a brief communication. *Exp Biol Med (Maywood).* 2003;228:967–71.

Berges RR, Windeler J, Trampisch HJ, et al. Randomised, placebo-controlled, double-blind clinical trial of beta-sitosterol in patients with benign prostatic hyperplasia. Beta-sitosterol Study Group. *Lancet.* 1995;345:1529–32.

Klippel KF, Hiltl DM, Schipp B. A multicentric, placebo-controlled, double-blind clinical trial of beta-sitosterol (phytosterol) for the treatment of benign prostatic hyperplasia. *Br J Urol.* 1997;80:427–32.

Wilt TJ, Ishani A, Stark G, et al. Saw palmetto extracts for treatment of benign prostatic hyperplasia: a systematic review. *JAMA.* 1998;280:1604–9.

Duffield-Lillico AJ, Dalkin BL, Reid ME, et al. Nutritional Prevention of Cancer Study Group. Selenium supplementation, baseline plasma selenium status and incidence of prostate cancer: an analysis of the complete treatment period of the Nutritional Prevention of Cancer Trial. *BJU Int.* 2003 May;91(7):608–12.

Chapter 5 (Sacral Chakra)

De Souza MC, Walker AF, Robinson PA, et al. A synergistic effect of a daily supplement for 1 month of 200 mg magnesium plus 50 mg vitamin B6 for the relief of anxiety-related premenstrual symptoms: a randomized, double-blind, crossover study. *J Womens Health Gend Based Med.* 2000;9:131–9.

Sharma P, Kulshreshtha S, Singh GM, et al. Role of bromocriptine and pyridoxine in premenstrual tension syndrome. *Indian J Physiol Pharmacol.* 2007 Oct–Dec; 51(4): 368–74.

Brush MG, Bennett T, Hansen K. Pyridoxine in the treatment of premenstrual syndrome: a retrospective survey in 630 patients. *Br J Clin Pract.* 1988 Nov;42(11):448–52.

Food and Nutrition Board, Institute of Medicine. *Dietary Reference Intakes for Vitamin C, Vitamin E, Selenium, and Carotenoids.* Washington, DC: National Academy Press, 2000. Available at: *books.nap.edu/0309069351/html/.*

Ward MW, Holimon TD. Calcium treatment for premenstrual syndrome. *Ann Pharmacother.* 1999 Dec;33(12):1356–8.

Bertone-Johnson ER, Hankinson SE, Bendich A, et al. Calcium and vitamin D intake and risk of incident premenstrual syndrome. *Arch Intern Med.* 2005 Jun 13;165(11): 1246–52.

Thys-Jacobs S, Ceccarelli S, Bierman A, et al. Calcium supplementation in premenstrual syndrome: a randomized crossover trial. *J Gen Intern Med.* 1989 May-Jun;4(3):183–9.

Facchinetti F, Borella P, Sances G, et al. Oral magnesium successfully relieves premenstrual mood changes. *Obstet Gynecol.* 1991;78:177–81.

Walker AF, De Souza MC, Vickers MF, et al. Magnesium supplementation alleviates premenstrual symptoms of fluid retention. *J Womens Health* 1998;7:1157–65.

Quaranta S, Buscaglia MA, Meroni MG, et al. Pilot study of the efficacy and safety of a modified-release magnesium 250 mg tablet (Sincromag) for the treatment of premenstrual syndrome. *Clin Drug Investig.* 2007;27(1):51–8.

Reid ME, Duffield-Lillico AJ, Slate E, et al. The nutritional prevention of cancer: 400 mcg per day selenium treatment. *Nutr Cancer.* 2008 Mar-Apr;60(2):155–63.

Hess MJ, Hess PE, Sullivan MR, et al. Evaluation of cranberry tablets for the prevention of urinary tract infections in spinal cord injured patients with neurogenic bladder. *Spinal Cord.* 2008 Sep;46(9):622-6. Epub 2008 Apr 8.

Minich DM, Bland JS. A review of the clinical efficacy and safety of cruciferous vegetable phytochemicals. *Nutr Rev.* 2007 Jun;65(6 Pt 1):259–67.

Bell MC, Crowley-Nowick P, Bradlow HL, et al. Placebo-controlled trial of indole-3-carbinol in the treatment of CIN. *Gynecol Oncol.* 2000;78:123–9.

van de Weijer P, Barentsen R. Isoflavones from red clover (Promensil) significantly reduce menopausal hot flush symptoms compared with placebo. *Maturitas.* 2002;42:187-93.

Nelsen J, Barrette E, Tsouronix C, et al. Red clover *(Trifolium pratense)* monograph: A clinical decision support tool. *J Herb Pharmacother.* 2002;2:49-72.

Gerli S, Papaleo E, Ferrari A, et al. Randomized, double blind placebo-controlled trial: effects of myo-inositol on ovarian function and metabolic factors in women with PCOS. *Eur Rev Med Pharmacol Sci.* 2007 Sep-Oct;11(5):347-54.

Chew BP, Wong MW, Park JS, et al. Dietary beta-carotene and astaxanthin but not can-thaxanthin stimulate splenocyte function in mice. *Anticancer Res.* 1999;19;5223-8.

Chapter 6 (Solar Plexus Chakra)

Food and Nutrition Board, Institute of Medicine. *Dietary Reference Intakes for Thiamin, Riboflavin, Niacin, Vitamin B6, Folate, Vitamin B12, Pantothenic Acid, Biotin, and Cho-line.* Washington, DC: National Academy Press, 2000. Available at: *books.nap. edu/0309065542/html/*

Althius MD, Jordon NE, Ludington EA, et al. Glucose and insulin responses to dietary chromium supplements: a meta-analysis. *Am J Clin Nutr.* 2002;76:148–55.

Anton SD, Morrison CD, Cefalu WT, et al. Effects of chromium picolinate on food intake and satiety. *Diabetes Technol Ther.* 2008 Oct;10(5):405–12.

Konrad T, Vicini P, Kusterer K, et al. Alpha-lipoic acid treatment decreases serum lac-tate and pyruvate concentrations and improves glucose effectiveness in lean and obese patients with Type 2 diabetes. *Diabetes Care.* 1999;22:280–7.

Kamenova P. Improvement of insulin sensitivity in patients with type 2 diabetes mel-litus after oral administration of alpha-lipoic acid. *Hormones (Athens).* 2006 Oct-Dec;5(4):251–8.

Jacob S, Ruus P, Hermann R, et al. Oral administration of RAC-alpha-lipoic acid modulates insulin sensitivity in patients with type-2 diabetes mellitus: a placebo-controlled pilot trial. *Free Radic Biol Med.* 1999 Aug;27(3-4):309–14.

Khan A, Safdar M, Ali Khan M, et al. Cinnamon improves glucose and lipids of people with type 2 diabetes. *Diabetes Care.* 2003;26:3215–8.

Momordica charantia (bitter melon). Monograph. *Altern Med Rev.* 2007 Dec;12(4):360–3.

Madar Z, Abel R, Samish S, et al. Glucose-lowering effect of fenugreek in non-insulin dependent diabetics. *Eur J Clin Nutr.* 1988;42:51–4.

Gupta A, Gupta R, Lal B. Effect of *Trigonella foenum-graecum* (fenugreek) seeds on gly-caemic control and insulin resistance in type 2 diabetes mellitus: a double blind placebo controlled study. *J Assoc Physicians India.* 2001;49:1057–61.

Shanmugasundaram ER, Rajeswari G, Baskaran K, et al. Use of *Gymnema sylvestre* leaf extract in the control of blood glucose in insulin-dependent diabetes mellitus. *J Ethnopharmacol.* 1990;30:281–94.

Baskaran K, Kizar-Ahamath B, Shanmugasundaram MR, et al. Antidiabetic effect of leaf extract from *Gymnema sylvestre* in non-insulin-dependent diabetes mellitus patients. *J Ethnopharmacol.* 1990;30:295–300.

Gymnema sylvestre. Altern Med Rev. 1999 Feb;4(1):46–7.

Vuksan V, Sievenpiper JL, Koo VY, et al. American ginseng *(Panax quinquefolius L)* reduces postprandial glycemia in nondiabetic subjects and subjects with type 2 diabetes mellitus. *Arch Intern Med.* 2000;160:1009–13.

Fischer-Rasmussen W, Kjaer SK, Dahl C, et al. Ginger treatment of hyperemesis gravidarum. *Eur J Obstet Gynecol Reprod Biol.* 1991;38:19–24.

Pongrojpaw D, Somprasit C, Chanthasenanont A. A randomized comparison of ginger and dimenhydrinate in the treatment of nausea and vomiting in pregnancy. *J Med Assoc Thai.* 2007;90:1703–9.

Wu KL, Rayner CK, Chuah SK, et al. Effects of ginger on gastric emptying and motility in healthy humans. *Eur J Gastroenterol Hepatol.* 2008 May;20(5):436–40.

Gonlachanvit S, Chen YH, Hasler WL, et al. Ginger reduces hyperglycemia-evoked gastric dysrhythmias in healthy humans: possible role of endogenous prostaglandins. *J Pharmacol Exp Ther.* 2003 Dec;307(3):1098-103. Epub 2003 Oct 8.

Prucksunand C, Indrasukhsri B, Leethochawalit M, et al. Phase II clinical trial on effect of the long turmeric *(Curcuma longa Linn)* on healing of peptic ulcer. *Southeast Asian J Trop Med Public Health.* 2001 Mar;32(1):208–15.

Thamlikitkul V, Bunyapraphatsara N, Dechatiwongse T, et al. Randomized double blind study of *Curcuma domestica Val.* for dyspepsia. *J Med Assoc Thai.* 1989;72:613–20.

Yates AA, Schlicker SA, Suitor CW. Dietary reference intakes: The new basis for recommendations for calcium and related nutrients, B vitamins, and choline. *J Am Diet Assoc.* 1998;98:699–706.

Ferenci P, Dragosics B, Dittrich H, et al. Randomized controlled trial of silymarin treatment in patients with cirrhosis of the liver. *J Hepatol.* 1989;9:105–13.

Buzzelli G, Moscarella S, Giusti A, et al. A pilot study on the liver protective effect of silybin-phosphatidylcholine complex (IdB1016) in chronic active hepatitis. *Int J Clin Pharmacol Ther Toxicol.* 1993;31:456–60.

Malaguarnera M, Cammalleri L, Gargante MP, et al. L-Carnitine treatment reduces severity of physical and mental fatigue and increases cognitive functions in centenarians: a randomized and controlled clinical trial. *Am J Clin Nutr.* 2007;86:1738–44.

Dulloo AG, Duret C, Rohrer D, et al. Efficacy of a green tea extract rich in catechin polyphenols and caffeine in increasing 24-h energy expenditure and fat oxidation in humans. *Am J Clin Nutr.* 1999;70:1040–5.

Zheng G, Sayama K, Okubo T, et al. Anti-obesity effects of three major components of green tea, catechins, caffeine and theanine, in mice. *In Vivo.* 2004;18:55–62.

Venables MC, Hulston CJ, Cox HR, et al. Green tea extract ingestion, fat oxidation, and glucose tolerance in healthy humans. *Am J Clin Nutr.* 2008 Mar;87(3):778–84.

Boschmann M, Thielecke F. The effects of epigallocatechin-3-gallate on thermogenesis and fat oxidation in obese men: a pilot study. *J Am Coll Nutr.* 2007 Aug;26(4):389S–395S.

Chapter 7 (Heart Chakra)

Hambrecht R, Hilbrich L, Erbs S, et al. Correction of endothelial dysfunction in chronic heart failure: additional effects of exercise training and oral L-arginine supplementation. *J Am Coll Cardiol.* 2000;35:706–13.

Rector TS, Bank AJ, Mullen KA, et al. Randomized, double-blind, placebo-controlled study of supplemental oral L-arginine in patients with heart failure. *Circulation.* 1996;93:2135–41.

Anderson JW, Johnstone BM, Cook-Newell ME. Meta-analysis of the effects of soy protein intake on serum lipids. *N Engl J Med.* 1995;333:276–82.

van der Griend R, Biesma DH, Haas FJLM, et al. The effect of different treatment regimens in reducing fasting and postmethionine-load homocysteine concentrations. *J Int Med.* 2000;248:223–9.

van der Griend R, Haas FJ, Biesma DH, et al. Combination of low-dose folic acid and pyridoxine for treatment of hyperhomocysteinaemia in patients with premature arterial disease and their relatives. *Atherosclerosis.* 1999;143:177–83.

Cheung AM, Tile L, Lee Y, et al. Vitamin K supplementation in postmenopausal women with osteopenia (ECKO trial): a randomized controlled trial. *PLoS Med.* 2008 Oct 14;5(10):e196.

van Summeren MJ, Braam LA, Lilien MR, et al. The effect of menaquinone-7 (vitamin K2) supplementation on osteocalcin carboxylation in healthy prepubertal children. *Br J Nutr.* 2009 May 19:1–8. [Epub ahead of print]

Shea MK, O'Donnell CJ, Hoffmann U, et al. Vitamin K supplementation and progression of coronary artery calcium in older men and women. *Am J Clin Nutr.* 2009 Jun;89(6):1799–807. Epub 2009 Apr 22.

Patrick L. Iodine: deficiency and therapeutic considerations. *Altern Med Rev.* 2008 Jun;13(2):116–27.

Ghent WR, Eskin BA, Low DA, et al. Iodine replacement in fibrocystic disease of the breast. *Can J Surg.* 1993;36:453–60.

Sanjuliani AF, de Abreu Fagundes VG, Francischetti EA. Effects of magnesium on blood pressure and intracellular ion levels of Brazilian hypertensive patients. *Int J Cardiol.* 1996;56:177–83.

Widman L, Wester PO, Stegmayr BK, et al. The dose-dependent reduction in blood pressure through administration of magnesium. A double blind placebo controlled cross-over study. *Am J Hypertens.* 1993;6:41–5.

Jee SH, Miller ER 3rd, Guallar E, et al. The effect of magnesium supplementation on blood pressure: a meta-analysis of randomized clinical trials. *Am J Hypertens.* 2002;15:691–6.

Guerrero-Romero F, Rodríguez-Morán M. The effect of lowering blood pressure by magnesium supplementation in diabetic hypertensive adults with low serum magnesium levels: a randomized, double-blind, placebo-controlled clinical trial. *J Hum Hypertens.* 2008 Nov 20. [Epub ahead of print.]

Food and Drug Administration. FDA Talk Paper: FDA Authorizes New Coronary Heart Disease Health Claim for Plant Sterol and Plant Stanol Esters. September 5, 2000. Accessed 21 Nov. 2009 at *www.fda.gov/bbs/topics/answers/ans01033.html.*

Heber D, Yip I, Ashley JM, et al. Cholesterol-lowering effects of a proprietary Chinese red-yeast-rice dietary supplement. *Am J Clin Nutr.* 1999;69:231–6.

Huang CF, Li TC, Lin CC, et al. Efficacy of Monascus purpureus Went rice on lowering lipid ratios in hypercholesterolemic patients. *Eur J Cardiovasc Prev Rehabil.* 2007 Jun;14(3):438–40.

Anonymous. Quercetin. *Alt Med Rev.* 1998;3:140–3.

Edwards RL, Lyon T, Litwin SE et al. Quercetin reduces blood pressure in hypertensive subjects. *J Nutr.* 2007 Nov;137(11):2405–11.

Belcaro G, Cesarone MR, Ledda A, et al. 5-year control and treatment of edema and increased capillary filtration in venous hypertension and diabetic microangiopathy using O-(beta-hydroxyethyl)-rutosides: a prospective comparative clinical registry. *Angiology.* 2008 Feb-Mar;59 Suppl 1:14S–20S.

Ried K, Frank OR, Stocks NP, et al. Effect of garlic on blood pressure: A systematic review and meta-analysis. *BMC Cardiovasc Disord.* 2008;8:13.

Koscielny J, Klüssendorf D, Latza R, et al. The antiatherosclerotic effect of *Allium sativum. Atherosclerosis.* 1999;144:237–49.

De Sanctis MT, Belcaro G, Incandela L, et al. Treatment of edema and increased capillary filtration in venous hypertension with total triterpenic fraction of *Centella asiatica:* a clinical, prospective, placebo-controlled, randomized, dose-ranging trial. *Angiology.* 2001;52 Suppl 2:S55–9.

Suter A, Bommer S, Rechner J. Treatment of patients with venous insufficiency with fresh plant horse chestnut seed extract: a review of 5 clinical studies. *Adv Ther.* 2006 Jan-Feb;23(1):179–90.

Tauchert M. Efficacy and safety of crataegus extract WS 1442 in comparison with placebo in patients with chronic stable New York Heart Association class-III heart failure. *Am Heart J.* 2002;143:910–5.

Holubarsch CJ, Colucci WS, Meinertz T, et al. The efficacy and safety of Crataegus extract WS(R) 1442 in patients with heart failure: The SPICE trial. *Eur J Heart Fail.* 2008 Nov 17. [Epub ahead of print.]

Sesso HD, Buring JE, Norkus EP, et al. Plasma lycopene, other carotenoids, and retinol and the risk of cardiovascular disease in women. *Am J Clin Nutr.* 2004 Jan;79(1):47–53.

Sesso HD, Liu S, Gaziano JM, et al. Dietary lycopene, tomato-based food products and cardiovascular disease in women. *J Nutr.* 2003;133:2336–41.

Neuman I, Nahum H, Ben-Amotz A. Reduction of exercise-induced asthma oxidative stress by lycopene, a natural antioxidant. *Allergy.* 2000;55:1184–9.

Chapter 8 (Throat Chakra)

Patrick L. Iodine: deficiency and therapeutic considerations. *Altern Med Rev.* 2008 Jun;13(2):116–27.

Mazokopakis EE, Papadakis JA, Papadomanolaki MG, et al. Effects of 12 months treatment with L-selenomethionine on serum anti-TPO levels in patients with Hashimoto's thyroiditis. *Thyroid.* 2007 Jul;17(7):609–12.

Allergic sinusitis. MedlinePlus Medical Encyclopedia. Accessed at: *www.nlm.nih.gov/medlineplus/ency/article/000813.htm.*

Thornhill SM, Kelly AM. Natural treatment of perennial allergic rhinitis. *Altern Med Rev.* 2000 Oct;5(5):448–54.

Mao TK, Van de Water J, Gershwin ME. Effects of a spirulina-based dietary supplement on cytokine production from allergic rhinitis patients. *J Med Food.* 2005;8:27-30.

Mittman P. Randomized, double-blind study of freeze-dried *Urtica dioica* in the treatment of allergic rhinitis. *Planta Med.* 1990;56:44–7.

Barrager E, Veltmann JR Jr, Schauss AG, Schiller RN. A multicentered, open-label trial on the safety and efficacy of methylsulfonylmethane in the treatment of seasonal allergic rhinitis. *J Altern Complement Med.* 2002 Apr;8(2):167–73.

Thie NM, Prasad NG, Major PW. Evaluation of glucosamine sulfate compared to ibuprofen for the treatment of temporomandibular joint osteoarthritis: a randomized double blind controlled 3 month clinical trial. *J Rheumatol.* 2001;28:1347–55.

Attias J, Weisz G, Almog S, et al. Oral magnesium intake reduces permanent hearing loss induced by noise exposure. *Am J Otolaryngol.* 1994 Jan-Feb;15(1):26–32.

Heyneman CA. Zinc deficiency and taste disorders. *Ann Pharmacother.* 1996;30:186–7.

Chapter 9 (Third Eye Chakra)

Emsley R, Myburgh C, Oosthuizen P, et al. Randomized, placebo-controlled study of ethyl-eicosapentaenoic acid as supplemental treatment in schizophrenia. *Am J Psychiatry.* 2002;159:1596–8.

Joy CB, Mumby-Croft R, Joy LA. Polyunsaturated fatty acid supplementation for schizophrenia. *Cochrane Database Syst Rev.* 2006;3:CD001257.

Zanarini MC, Frankenburg FR. Omega-3 fatty acid treatment of women with borderline personality disorder: a double-blind, placebo-controlled pilot study. *Am J Psychiatry.* 2003;160:167–9.

Sivrioglu EY, Kirli S, Sipahioglu D, et al. The impact of omega-3 fatty acids, vitamins E and C supplementation on treatment outcome and side effects in schizophrenia patients treated with haloperidol: an open-label pilot study. *Prog Neuropsychopharmacol Biol Psychiatry.* 2007 Oct 1;31(7):1493-9. Epub 2007 Jul 13.

Malcolm CA, McCulloch DL, Montgomery C, et al. Maternal docosahexaenoic acid supplementation during pregnancy and visual evoked potential development in term infants: a double blind, prospective, randomised trial. *Arch Dis Child Fetal Neonatal Ed.* 2003;88:F383–90.

Stordy BJ. Dark adaptation, motor skills, docosahexaenoic acid, and dyslexia. *Am J Clin Nutr.* 2000;71:323S–6S.

Lerner V, Miodownik C, Kaptsan A, et al. Vitamin B6 as add-on treatment in chronic schizophrenic and schizoaffective patients: a double-blind, placebo-controlled study. *J Clin Psychiatry.* 2002 Jan;63(1):54–8.

Wyatt KM, Dimmock PW, Jones PW, et al. Efficacy of vitamin B-6 in the treatment of premenstrual syndrome: systematic review. *BMJ.* 1999 May 22;318(7195):1375–81.

Hvas AM, Juul S, Bech P, et al. Vitamin B6 level is associated with symptoms of depression. *Psychother Psychosom.* 2004 Nov-Dec;73(6):340–3.

Kuzminski AM, Del Giacco EJ, Allen RH, et al. Effective treatment of cobalamin deficiency with oral cobalamin. *Blood.* 1998;92:1191–8.

Andres E, Kurtz JE, Perrin AE, et al. Oral cobalamin therapy for the treatment of patients with food-cobalamin malabsorption. *Am J Med.* 2001;111:126–9.

Wald DS, Bishop L, Wald NJ, et al. Randomized trial of folic acid supplementation and serum homocysteine levels. *Arch Intern Med.* 2001;161:695–700.

Kendrick T, Dunn N, Robinson S, et al. A longitudinal study of blood folate levels and depressive symptoms among young women in the Southampton Women's Survey. *J Epidemiol Community Health.* 2008 Nov;62(11):966–72.

Tolmunen T, Hintikka J, Voutilainen S, et al. Association between depressive symptoms and serum concentrations of homocysteine in men: a population study. *Am J Clin Nutr.* 2004 Dec;80(6):1574–8.

Homocysteine Lowering Trialists' Collaboration. Dose-dependent effects of folic acid on blood concentrations of homocysteine: a meta-analysis of the randomized trials. *Am J Clin Nutr.* 2005 Oct;82(4):806–12.

Young SN. Folate and depression—a neglected problem. *J Psychiatry Neurosci.* 2007 Mar;32(2):80–2.

Cooper JR. The role of ascorbic acid in the oxidation of tryptophan to 5-hydroxytryptophan. *Ann NY Acad Sci.* 1961;92:208–11.

Milner G. Ascorbic acid in chronic psychiatric patients: a controlled trial. *Br J Psychiatry.* 1963;109:294–9.

Dakhale GN, Khanzode SD, Khanzode SS, et al. Supplementation of vitamin C with atypical antipsychotics reduces oxidative stress and improves the outcome of schizophrenia. *Psychopharmacology (Berl).* 2005 Nov;182(4):494-8. Epub 2005 Oct 19.

Sivrioglu EY, Kirli S, Sipahioglu D, et al. The impact of omega-3 fatty acids, vitamins E and C supplementation on treatment outcome and side effects in schizophrenia patients treated with haloperidol: an open-label pilot study. *Prog Neuropsychopharmacol Biol Psychiatry.* 2007 Oct 1;31(7):1493–9. Epub 2007 Jul 13.

Przybelski RJ, Binkley NC. Is vitamin D important for preserving cognition? A positive correlation of serum 25-hydroxyvitamin D concentration with cognitive function. *Arch Biochem Biophys.* 2007 Apr 15;460(2):202–5. Epub 2007 Jan 8.

Johnson MA, Fischer JG, Park S. Vitamin D deficiency and insufficiency in the Georgia Older Americans Nutrition Program. *J Nutr Elder.* 2008;27(1-2):29–46.

Jorde R, Sneve M, Figenschau Y, et al. Effects of vitamin D supplementation on symptoms of depression in overweight and obese subjects: randomized double blind trial. *J Intern Med.* 2008 Dec 1;264(6):599–609. Epub 2008 Sep 10.

Hoogendijk WJ, Lips P, Dik MG, et al. Depression is associated with decreased 25-hydroxyvitamin D and increased parathyroid hormone levels in older adults. *Arch Gen Psychiatry.* 2008 May;65(5):508–12.

Wilkins CH, Sheline YI, Roe CM, et al. Vitamin D deficiency is associated with low mood and worse cognitive performance in older adults. *Am J Geriatr Psychiatry.* 2006 Dec;14(12):1032–40.

Brown D, Gaby A., and Reichert R. Altering the Brain's Chemistry to Elevate Mood. Accessed at *www.healthyplace.com/COMMUNITIES/depression/treatment/alterntive/brain_chemistry.asp.*

Siwek M, Wróbel A, Dudek D, et al. [The role of copper and magnesium in the pathogenesis and treatment of affective disorders]. [Article in Polish]. *Psychiatr Pol.* 2005 Sep-Oct;39(5):911–20.

Peikert A, Wilimzig C, Kohne-Volland R. Prophylaxis of migraine with oral magnesium: results from a prospective, multi-center, placebo-controlled and double-blind randomized study. *Cephalalgia.* 1996;16:257–63.

Held K, Antonijevic IA, Künzel H, et al. Oral Mg(2+) supplementation reverses age-related neuroendocrine and sleep EEG changes in humans. *Pharmacopsychiatry.* 2002 Jul;35(4):135–43.

Thal LJ, Carta A, Clarke WR, et al. A 1-year multicenter placebo-controlled study of acetyl-L-carnitine in patients with Alzheimer's Disease. *Neurology.* 1996;47: 705–11.

Sano M, Bell K, Cote L, et al. Double-blind parallel design pilot study of acetyl levocarnitine in patients with Alzheimer's Disease. *Arch Neurol.* 1992;49:1137-41.

Rai G, Wright G, Scott L, et al. Double-blind, placebo controlled study of acetyl-l-carnitine in patients with Alzheimer's dementia. *Curr Med Res Opin.* 1990;11: 638–47.

Nakajima T, Kudo Y, Kaneko Z. Clinical evaluation of 5-hydroxy-L-tryptophan as an antidepressant drug. *Folia Psychiatr Neurol Jpn.* 1978;32:223–30.

Levine J, Barak Y, Gonzalves M, et al. Double-blind, controlled trial of inositol treatment of depression. *Am J Psychiatry.* 1995;152:792–4.

Benjamin J, Levine J, Fux M, et al. Double-blind, placebo-controlled, crossover trial of inositol treatment for panic disorder. *Am J Psychiatry.* 1995;152:1084–6.

Palatnik A, Frolov K, Fux M, et al. Double-blind, controlled, crossover trial of inositol versus fluvoxamine for the treatment of panic disorder. *J Clin Psychopharmacol.* 2001;21:335–9.

Fux M, Levine J, Aviv A, et al. Inositol treatment of obsessive-compulsive disorder. *Am J Psychiatry.* 1996;153:1219–21.

Kim HL, Streltzer J, Goebert D. St. John's wort for depression: a meta analysis of well-defined clinical trials. *J Nerv Ment Dis.* 1999;187:532–9.

Linde K, Ramirez G, Mulrow CD, et al. St. John's wort for depression: an overview and meta-analysis of randomized clinical trials. *BMJ.* 1996;313:253–8.

Zhdanova IV, Wurtman RJ, Regan MM, et al. Melatonin treatment for age-related insomnia. *J Clin Endocrinol Metab.* 2001;86:4727–30.

Brusco LI, Fainstein I, Marquez M, et al. Effect of melatonin in selected populations of sleep-disturbed patients. *Biol Signals Recept.* 1999;8:126–31.

Dorn M. [Efficacy and tolerability of Baldrian versus oxazepam in non-organic and non-psychiatric insomniacs: a randomized, double-blind, clinical, comparative study]. [Article in German]. *Forsch Komplementarmed Klass Naturheilkd.* 2000;7:79–84.

Bent S, Padula A, Moore D, et al. Valerian for sleep: a systematic review and meta-analysis. *Am J Med.* 2006 Dec;119(12):1005–12.

Richer S, Stiles W, Statkute L, et al. Double-masked, placebo-controlled, randomized trial of lutein and antioxidant supplementation in the intervention of atrophic age-related macular degermation: the Veterans LAST study (Lutein Antioxidant Supplement Trial). *Optometry.* 2004;75:216–30.

Bahrami H, Melia M, Dagnelie G. Lutein supplementation in retinitis pigmentosa: PC-based vision assessment in a randomized double-masked placebo-controlled clinical trial [NCT00029289]. *BMC Ophthalmol.* 2006 Jun 7;6:23.

Olmedilla B, Granado F, Blanco I, et al. Lutein, but not alpha-tocopherol, supplementation improves visual function in patients with age-related cataracts: a 2-y double-blind, placebo-controlled pilot study. *Nutrition.* 2003 Jan;19(1):21–4.

Stough C, Lloyd J, Clarke J, et al. The chronic effects of an extract of *Bacopa monniera* (Brahmi) on cognitive function in healthy human subjects. *Psychopharmacology.* 2001;156:481–4.

Stough C, Downey LA, Lloyd J, et al. Examining the nootropic effects of a special extract of *Bacopa monniera* on human cognitive functioning: 90 day double-blind placebo-controlled randomized trial. *Phytother Res.* 2008 Aug 6. [Epub ahead of print.]

Wattanathorn J, Mator L, Muchimapura S, et al. Positive modulation of cognition and mood in the healthy elderly volunteer following the administration of *Centella asiatica. J Ethnopharmacol.* 2008 Mar 5;116(2):325-32. Epub 2007 Dec 4.

Crook T, Petrie W, Wells C, Massari DC. Effects of phosphatidylserine in Alzheimer's disease. *Psychopharmacol Bull.* 1992;28:61–6.

Delwaide PJ, Gyselynck-Mambourg AM, Hurlet A, Ylieff M. Double-blind, randomized, controlled study of phosphatidylserine in senile demented patients. *Acta Neurol Scand.* 1986;73:136–40.

Schreiber S, Kampf-Sherf O, Gorfine M, et al. An open trial of plant-source derived phosphatidylserine for treatment of age-related cognitive decline. *Isr J Psychiatry Relat Sci.* 2000;37:302–7.

Kelly SP, Gomez-Ramirez M, Montesi JL, et al. L-theanine and caffeine in combination affect human cognition as evidenced by oscillatory alpha-band activity and attention task performance. *J Nutr.* 2008 Aug;138(8):1572S–1577S.

Gomez-Ramirez M, Kelly SP, Montesi JL, et al. The Effects of L-theanine on Alpha-Band Oscillatory Brain Activity During a Visuo-Spatial Attention Task. *Brain Topogr.* 2008 Oct 9. [Epub ahead of print]

Chapter 10 (Crown Chakra)

Jamal GA, Carmichael H. The effect of gamma-linolenic acid on human diabetic peripheral neuropathy: a double-blind placebo-controlled trial. *Diabet Med.* 1990;7: 319–23.

Keen H, Payan J, Allawi J, et al. Treatment of diabetic neuropathy with gamma-linolenic acid. The Gamma-Linolenic Acid Multicenter Trial Group. *Diabetes Care.* 1993;16:8–15.

Okuda Y, Mizutani M, Ogawa M, et al. Long-term effects of eicosapentaenoic acid on diabetic peripheral neuropathy and serum lipids in patients with type II diabetes mellitus. *J Diabetes Complications.* 1996 Sep-Oct;10(5):280–7.

Gerbi A, Maixent JM, Ansaldi JL, et al. Fish oil supplementation prevents diabetes-induced nerve conduction velocity and neuroanatomical changes in rats. *J Nutr.* 1999 Jan;129(1):207–13.

Koutsikos D, Agroyannis B, Tzanatos-Exarchou H. Biotin for diabetic peripheral neuropathy. *Biomed Pharmacother.* 1990;44(10):511–4.

Haupt E, Ledermann H, Köpcke W. Benfotiamine in the treatment of diabetic polyneuropathy—a three-week randomized, controlled pilot study (BEDIP study). *Int J Clin Pharmacol Ther.* 2005 Feb;43(2):71–7.

Scalabrino G, Peracchi M. New insights into the pathophysiology of cobalamin deficiency. *Trends Mol Med.* 2006 Jun;12(6):247-54. Epub 2006 May 11.

Head KA. Peripheral neuropathy: pathogenic mechanisms and alternative therapies. *Altern Med Rev.* 2006 Dec;11(4):294–329.

Tütüncü NB, Bayraktar M, Varli K. Reversal of defective nerve conduction with vitamin E supplementation in type 2 diabetes: a preliminary study. *Diabetes Care.* 1998 Nov;21(11):1915–8.

De Leeuw I, Engelen W, De Block C, et al. Long term magnesium supplementation influences favourably the natural evolution of neuropathy in Mg-depleted type 1 diabetic patients (T1dm). *Magnes Res.* 2004 Jun;17(2):109–14.

Calabrese V, Scapagnini G, Ravagna A, Bella R, Butterfield DA, Calvani M, Pennisi G, Giuffrida Stella AM. Disruption of thiol homeostasis and nitrosative stress in the cerebrospinal fluid of patients with active multiple sclerosis: evidence for a protective role of acetylcarnitine. *Neurochem Res.* 2003 Sep;28(9):1321–8.

De Grandis D, Minardi C. Acetyl-L-carnitine (levacecarnine) in the treatment of diabetic neuropathy. A long-term, randomised, double-blind, placebo-controlled study. *Drugs R D.* 2002;3:223–31.

Sima AAF, Calvani M, Mehra M, et al. Acetyl-L-carnitine improves pain, nerve regeneration, and vibratory perception in patients with chronic diabetic neuropathy: an analysis of two randomized, placebo-controlled trials. *Diabetes Care.* 2005;28: 89–94.

Ziegler D, Hanefeld M, Ruhnau K, et al. Treatment of symptomatic diabetic polyneuropathy with the antioxidant alpha-lipoic acid: A 7-month, multicenter, randomized, controlled trial (ALADIN III Study). *Diabetes Care.* 1999;22:1296–301.

Reljanovic M, Reichel G, Rett K, et al. Treatment of diabetic polyneuropathy with the antioxidant thioctic acid (alpha-lipoic acid): a 2-year, multicenter, randomized, double-blind, placebo-controlled trial (ALADIN II). Alpha Lipoic Acid in Diabetic Neuropathy. *Free Radic Res.* 1999;31:171–7.

Ruhnau KJ, Meissner HP, Finn JR, et al. Effects of 3-week oral treatment with the antioxidant thioctic acid (alpha-lipoic acid) in symptomatic diabetic polyneuropathy. *Diabet Med.* 1999;16:1040–3.

Shults CW, Oakes D, Kieburtz K, et al. Effects of coenzyme Q10 in early Parkinson disease: evidence of slowing of the functional decline. *Arch Neurol.* 2002;59: 1541–50.

Yates AA, Schlicker SA, Suitor CW. Dietary reference intakes: The new basis for recommendations for calcium and related nutrients, B vitamins, and choline. *J Am Diet Assoc.* 1998;98:699–706.

Sima AA, Dunlap JA, Davidson EP, et al. Supplemental myo-inositol prevents L-fucose-induced diabetic neuropathy. *Diabetes.* 1997 Feb;46(2):301–6.

Sundkvist G, Dahlin LB, Nilsson H, et al. Sorbitol and myo-inositol levels and morphology of sural nerve in relation to peripheral nerve function and clinical neuropathy in men with diabetic, impaired, and normal glucose tolerance. *Diabet Med.* 2000 Apr;17(4):259–68.

Bourre JM. Effects of nutrients (in food) on the structure and function of the nervous system: update on dietary requirements for brain. Part 1: micronutrients. *J Nutr Health Aging.* 2006 Sep-Oct;10(5):377–85.

Zeisel SH. Choline: needed for normal development of memory. *J Am Coll Nutr.* 2000;19:528S–31S.

Shaw GM, Carmichael SL, Yang W, et al. Periconceptional dietary intake of choline and betaine and neural tube defects in offspring. *Am J Epidemiol.* 2004;160:102–9.

GLOSSARY

Adaptogens: Substances (typically herbs) that have a balancing effect on the body's reactions to stress (e.g., *Eleutherococcus senticosus*).

Alkaloids: Natural compounds that can have strong physiological effects. Can also be potentially toxic.

Alpha-linolenic acid: Omega-3 fat from nonanimal sources (green vegetables, seeds, and nuts). Can be metabolized in the body to form other omega-3 fats that have specific functions, such as eicosapentaenoic acid (EPA) and docosahexaenoic acid (DHA).

Amino acids: Building blocks of protein. Select amino acids are metabolized to neurotransmitters (e.g., tryptophan is metabolized to serotonin).

Antioxidant: Compound that protects cells from damage by reactive chemical groups. May be water soluble (e.g., vitamin C) or fat soluble (e.g., vitamin E).

Anthocyanidins: A class of purple-colored plant pigments that act as antioxidants, particularly in the central nervous system.

Bioflavonoids: A class of compounds found in plant sources, especially citrus fruits. Common bioflavonoids include quercetin and rutin.

Carbohydrate: Macronutrient found in foods and supplements. Consists of carbon, hydrogen, and oxygen. Provides 4 calories per gram and a source of readily available energy. Includes simple sugars like glucose, more complex sugars like starches, and insoluble and soluble fibers.

Carotenoids: Family of plant compounds that often impart a particular color, such as red, orange or yellow. Some carotenoids, such as beta-carotene, can be converted in the body to vitamin A.

Cellulose: Insoluble plant fiber.

Chakra: Sanskrit word for "wheel." Refers to the wheel-like energy centers that direct subtle-energy flow in the body. There are seven main chakras, located mainly along the spine.

Crown chakra: Energy center responsible for divinity, interconnection, purity, universal truth. Vibrates at the same frequencies as the colors lavender and white. Resides at the top of the head.

Decoction: Method of preparing herbs for medicinal use. Involves the extraction of compounds through the process of making tea.

Detoxification: The process of clearing toxins from the body.

Dietary Reference Intakes (DRI):
Guidelines for nutrient intake established between 1997 and 2001 by the Food and Nutrition Board of the Institute of Medicine.

Dietary supplements: Additional nutritional support (sometimes in amounts greater than would be obtained from food alone) that can come in the form of macronutrients (carbohydrate, protein, fat), micronutrients (vitamins, minerals), and/or herbs.

Diuretic: Substance that encourages urination when ingested.

Docosahexaenoic acid (DHA):
Omega-3 fat derived from algae and fish sources. Important for brain, eye, and heart function.

Dysglycemia: Unhealthy handling of glucose (sugar) by the body, resulting in abnormal blood-glucose levels.

Eicosapentaenoic acid (EPA):
Omega-3 fat from fish sources. Has anti-inflammatory effects in the human body.

Essential fatty acids: Necessary fats that the human body cannot make on its own and must obtain from food sources (e.g., omega-3 fats from fish).

Extracellular matrix: Watery fluid that surrounds cells. Responsible for the transport of nutrients and waste products in and out of cells.

Extract (herbal): Method of distilling the active compounds in a plant using water or alcohol and then allowing the liquid to evaporate.

Fat: Macronutrient found in foods and supplements. Consists of carbon, hydrogen, and oxygen. Provides 9 calories per gram. Includes solid (generally animal) fats such as saturated fats, as well as liquid (typically vegetable) oils composed of primarily unsaturated fats. Performs several roles in the body, such as regulating hormones and maintaining a healthy heart and blood vessels, affecting moods and behavior, and protecting vision.

Fiber: Nondigestible form of carbohydrate. Passes through the intestinal tract without being absorbed and, thus, does not typically provide calories. (Note: some fibers are able to be fermented by gut bacteria and result in minimal calorie contribution.) Classified as either insoluble (does not swell in the presence of water) or soluble (swells in the presence of water; may result in better management of blood glucose and cholesterol).

Gamma-linolenic acid: Omega-6 fat from vegetarian sources (seeds, plants). Has anti-inflammatory activity in the human body.

HDL cholesterol: Referred to as "good" cholesterol since it clears cholesterol from tissues.

Heart chakra: Energy center responsible for love, emotional wisdom, compassion, giving, and receiving.

Connected to the color green. Resides in the middle of the upper torso, at the level of the physical heart organ, extending through the body to the upper-middle spine.

Homocysteine: Metabolic compound that has detrimental effects on the cardiovascular system when present in elevated amounts in the blood. Levels may be reduced with adequate intake of specific B vitamins.

Hydrogenation: A process that uses hydrogen to transform a liquid fat into a solid, shelf-stable fat.

Insoluble fiber: Fiber from plant sources (e.g., cellulose). Forms bulk in the intestine and thus may help with bowel movements.

Intrinsic factor: Protein in the stomach required for vitamin B12 absorption.

LDL cholesterol: Referred to as "bad" cholesterol since it is the primary transporter of cholesterol in the blood.

Leaky gut: Condition in which the intestine becomes too permeable, allowing for large, undigested particles to enter the blood.

Macronutrients: Nutrients that provide energy in the form of calories. Eaten in relatively large amounts (several grams) on a daily basis as part of the food supply (e.g., carbohydrate).

Methylation: The act of adding a chemical group called the methyl group, which is composed of a carbon atom and three hydrogen atoms, to a compound. Can have profound effects on the expression of genes.

Methylmercury: Organic form of mercury. Found in fish due to the contamination of ocean waters by mercury-containing waste.

Micronutrients: Substances that are needed in small quantities by the human body. Includes minerals and vitamins (e.g., zinc, vitamin B12).

Mineral: A solid crystalline structure that can be extracted from the earth's crust. The array of different minerals serves several functions within the human body (e.g., iron is needed to form hemoglobin, which ultimately helps oxygenate the body and provide energy to it).

Neurotransmitters: Chemicals made in the body that are exchanged between nerve cells (e.g., serotonin). Can produce overall changes in behavior, mood, thought, and memory.

Omega-3 fats: Essential fats that must be eaten in the diet that are usually liquid at room temperature. Obtained from algae, green vegetables, seeds, fish, and nuts. Important for specific functions in the human body, such as reducing inflammation and promoting healthy vision and brain function.

Omega-6 fats: Essential fats for the body that must be eaten in the diet. Sources include vegetables, nuts, and seeds. Required for specific functions in the human body, such as regulating hormone function and inflammation.

Phospholipids: Type of complex fat that has a phosphorus group as part of its structure. Typically found in cell membranes.

Phytoestrogens: Plant compound that acts like weak estrogen in the body.

Pigment: Colored compound found in plants.

Polyphenols: Plant compounds with antioxidant activity.

Prebiotics: Fibers that can be fermented by intestinal bacteria (e.g., inulin). The fermentation results in substances that keep healthy bacteria thriving in the gut.

Probiotics: Beneficial intestinal bacteria (e.g., *Lactobacillus acidophilus).*

Protein: Macronutrient made of amino acids. Provides calories (4 calories per gram), in addition to being used to form hormones, antibodies (immune cells), enzymes, and tissues.

Root chakra: Energy center responsible for trust, security, safety, and survival. Vibrates at the same frequencies as the color red. Resides below the level of the pubic bone and extends through the body to the tailbone (coccyx).

Sacral chakra: Energy center responsible for emotions, creativity, sexuality, and sensuality. Vibrates at the same frequencies as the color orange. Resides in the low abdomen under the navel, extending through the body to the sacrum.

Saturated fat: Fat mainly derived from animal sources. Tends to be solid at room temperature.

Sirtuins: Family of proteins that play a role in aging, metabolism, and longevity.

Solar plexus chakra: Energy center responsible for transformation, personal power, confidence, self-identity, and energy exchange. Vibrates at the same frequencies as the color yellow. Resides in the middle of the torso, under the diaphragm, and extends through the body to the middle spine.

Soluble fiber: Fiber obtained from fruits and other sources which swells in the presence of liquid (e.g., psyllium). Can assist in the slow release of glucose into the blood stream after a meal. May also trap dietary cholesterol and prevent its uptake in the body.

Third eye chakra: Energy center responsible for insight, imagination, wisdom, dreams, and psychic ability. Vibrates at the same frequencies as the colors indigo and violet. Resides in the middle of the forehead, between the eyes, and extends through the skull to the back of the head.

Throat chakra: Energy center responsible for truth, authenticity, communication, and surrender. Vibrates at the same frequencies as the color aquamarine. Resides in the throat area, extending through the body to the cervical spine.

Tincture (herbal): Plant constituents preserved in a liquid medium like alcohol or glycerin.

Tolerable upper limit (TUL): Upper level of nutrient intake (represents total intake from food, water, and supplements) considered to be safe and likely to pose no risk of side effects, as established by the Institute of Medicine. Amounts that exceed the upper limit may result in a greater propensity towards side effects.

Trans fats: Type of fat produced through the process of hydrogenation. Not considered to be heart healthy. Since 2006, the FDA requires food manufacturers to report the amount of trans fat in foods. If a food or supplement contains "partially hydrogenated oil," it contains some amount of trans fat. (Note: trans fats of a different type are found in small amounts in animal products like milk. These are not considered to have the same negative effects as those produced artificially.)

Unsaturated fat: Fat from vegetable sources. Liquid at room temperature. Omega-6 and omega-3 fats are examples of unsaturated fats.

Vitamin: Compound required by the human body in small amounts for a variety of functions (e.g., metabolism, synthesis of neurotransmitters, blood clotting). Not normally produced in the body; therefore, must be obtained from food or dietary supplements.

INDEX

ABOUT THE AUTHOR

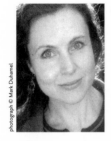

photograph © Mark Duhamel

Deanna Minich, Ph.D., C.N., *www.foodandspirit.com,* is a nutritionist who sees more to food than calories and macronutrients. She blends cutting-edge nutrition information, quantum physics, and the ancient chakra system to guide others to use foods and eating as tools for spiritual growth and nourishment for the soul. Her clinical practice using nutrition and dietary supplements along with transformative personal growth techniques has led her to create *Quantum Supplements,* as well as her other books, *Chakra Foods for Optimum Health: A Guide to the Foods that can Improve Your Energy, Inspire Creative Changes, Open Your Heart, and Heal Body, Mind, and Spirit* (Conari Press, 2009) and *An A–Z Guide to Food Additives: Never Eat What You Can't Pronounce* (Conari Press, 2009). The creative blend of science and spirituality she presents will open your heart, unravel your intuition, and guide you on a journey to inner and outer bliss with every bite you take!

Contact Dr. Minich at deannaminich@hotmail.com.

TO OUR READERS

Weiser Books, an imprint of Red Wheel/Weiser, publishes books across the entire spectrum of occult and esoteric subjects. Our mission is to publish quality books that will make a difference in people's lives without advocating any one particular path or field of study. We value the integrity, originality, and depth of knowledge of our authors.

Our readers are our most important resource, and we appreciate your input, suggestions, and ideas about what you would like to see published. Please feel free to contact us, to request our latest book catalog, or to be added to our mailing list.

Red Wheel/Weiser, LLC
500 Third Street, Suite 230
San Francisco, CA 94107
www.redwheelweiser.com